Go Vegan?

Review of Science

Part 1

By Milos Pokimica

Medical Disclaimer

The information provided in this book is just personal opinion of the author and is not intended or implied to be a substitute for professional medical advice, diagnosis or treatment. The information provided in this book is for informational purposes only and are not intended to serve as a substitute for the consultation, diagnosis, and/or medical treatment of a qualified physician or healthcare provider.

NEVER DISREGARD PROFESSIONAL MEDICAL ADVICE OR DELAY SEEKING MEDICAL TREATMENT BECAUSE OF SOMETHING YOU HAVE READ ON OR ACCESSED THROUGH THIS BOOK. NEVER APPLY ANY LIFESTYLE CHANGES OR ANY CHANGES AT ALL AS A CONSEQUENCE OF SOMETHING YOU HAVE READ IN THIS BOOK BEFOR CONSULTING LICENCED MEDICAL PRACTITIONER.

In the event of a medical emergency, call a doctor or 911 immediately. This book does not recommend or endorse any specific groups, organizations, tests, physicians, products, procedures, opinions, or other information that may be mentioned inside. Reliance on any information provided by this book is solely at your own risk.

None of the individual contributors, author, nor anyone else connected to this book can take any responsibility for the results or consequences of any attempt to use or adopt any of the information presented inside.

Warning:

This book contains images (which may be unsuitable for children and upsetting to adults) and topics and discussions which some readers might find upsetting.

Table of Contents:

Missing link?

"Know thyself"- Oracle of Delphi

What is the Missing Link? It is a non-scientific term for a nonexistent transitional fossil that is believed it would bridge the gap in evolution between higher apes and humans. Homo sapiens (Latin: "wise man") have a mutual ancestor with some other primate species. The hominid genetic family branch includes the group comprising of all modern and extinct great apes. That includes modern humans, gorillas, chimpanzees, and orangutans plus all of their direct ancestors. Hominins are a narrower term and include only those species that came after the human lineage split from that of chimpanzees. The lineage is ending with modern humans but also includes extinct human species and all of our immediate ancestors. It includes members of the species Homo, Paranthropus, Australopithecus, and Ardipithecus.

So what is the real missing link? It is the same gap in our logical understanding of how our body physiology came into fulfillment. What does that even mean? Well, it means something like this. If some species of the hominins are still alive today like Homo erectus, that evolved in Africa 1.9 million years ago, they will be so genetically similar to us that we will be able to engage into sexual intercourse with them and have mix marriages and children. Although children will probably be sterile like many other interspecies hybrids and would not be able to reproduce any further. We have a belief that somehow we are the smartest ones. We are better and more intelligent than all other primates and all other animals. With the use of fire and later technological inventions we have brought the rise of civilization. However, that is a lie. Archeological evidence demonstrates that the beginning of the controlled use of fire date back at some 650 thousand years ago by Homo erectus.

He had a wide range of other behaviors that we might "only" associate with anatomically modern humans. We are not even genetically pure Homo sapiens. We are a mixture of interbreeding between Homo sapiens and Neanderthal. Tibetans also have genes of Denisovans. It is a species that went extinct about 40,000 years ago. They inherited so-called a "super athlete" gene that helps Sherpas and other Tibetans breathe easy at high altitudes. It might be a strange idea to some people to think that we had been interbreeding with "primitive" species of primates but that is the truth. Those primitive wild primates are much more modern then we would like to think and still live in our genes. Rasmus Nielsen who specialized in the field of group genetics at the University of California, Berkeley, did some scientific research on the subject. Their team had studied the DNA samples and found that the Tibetans and in a smaller part, around 1 of the 20 Han Chinese had a unique segment of the EPAS1 gene. When they investigated the catalog of human genomes that was available in the 1000 Genomes Project, they could not find a match. Then, the team investigated the genes of archaic humans, including Neanderthals and a Denisovans. The Denisovan genome has previously been extracted and sequenced from the DNA in a finger bone that was discovered in Denisova Cave in the Altai Mountains of Siberia. The Tibetan and Denisovan gene segments matched. So how is it possible that the Tibetans have gotten this gene from these hominins? They have existed 40,000 years before them in Siberia and different sections of entire Asian continent. Nielsen and his research group employing computer modeling discovered that the only possible explanation was that the descendants of Tibetans got the gene by their ancestors mating with Denisovans. Recent genetic testing has also revealed that Melanesians in Papua New Guinea from all of the people on the planet have the highest levels of Denisovan DNA today. They have more than 5% of their entire genome inherited from Denisovans. Another team of researchers showed for example that Mayans in particular, have inherited one bad gene variant from Neanderthals. Even the ancestors of Native Americans had been interbreeding with Neanderthals. That gene variant today is creating a risk factor for type 2 diabetes in Mexico.

Now after all of this, we could say that genetically pure Homo sapiens does not even exist. Scientists will disagree with this statement, but it is true. Most of us have some genes inherited from Neanderthals or Denisovans or mixture of both. Now in regular science, they would say that although this is true the level of a mixture is not at the relevant level or in other words that genetic influx of Neanderthal genes is insignificant and that we are still in the genetic and physical form of regular Homo sapiens. I will admit that I do not have Ph.D. in this area of expertise but am pretty sure that 5% or 1 Denisovan on 19 humans plus some genes of Neanderthals is far from insignificant. Neanderthal and Denisovan genes still live in us, and not just in the form of anonymous DNA fragments but in the active part of our DNA. That part did not magically disappear. It remained in us and shapes the way we exist, and behave or what diseases or weaknesses we might have. The problem with this kind of data is psychological because of our underlying self-image. We consider ourselves to be above the rest of the hominid species and the rest of the species in general and the natural order. If for example I teach as a college professor and I would like to make a thesis that Melanesians in Papua New Guinea should get their new fancy Latin name instead of Homo sapiens, what would be the result? Why new name? Because they represent a form of hybrid of 5 % Denisovan 95% Homo sapiens. In cynology for example that will be considered a new type of dog breed. If I do that I would probably lose my job, won't be able to pay a mortgage, get labeled as racist and would be chased down the street by angry social justice warriors. The truth is that in science this had been known for a long time.

There were even some troublesome experiments done with the idea of making humanzee hybrids, a mix of chimpanzee and human. Chimpanzees and humans are closely related. We share about 95% of our DNA sequence and about 99% of coding DNA sequences, and that is the relatively small difference in biological terms. Because of this similarity, there was speculation that a hybrid could be feasible. Ilya Ivanovich Ivanov was the first scientist who had actually attempted to create a human-chimp hybrid. He tried to do this directly with artificial insemination. He proposed his idea back in 1910 in a presentation to the World Congress of Zoologists. However, he did not stop there. By the 1920s, he carried out a sequence of experiments with human sperm trying to inseminate female chimpanzees artificially. Luckily the experiment did not succeed, and he failed to achieve a successful pregnancy. However, that did not stop him, and by 1929 he prepared a set of experiments with nonhuman ape sperm and female human volunteers. Yes, he had female volunteers ready to be impregnated with the ape sperm. Luckily experiment was hindered by the death of his last orangutan. The next year when his experiments had become known to the public, he suffered strong condemnation from the Soviet government, and he was sentenced to exile. He operated briefly in the veterinary zoo-technical institute as an ordinary worker and did not do any more experiments, and two years later he died of a stroke. This kind of hybridization in nature is very plausible and had already been done by large extent to increase the profits in the food business. Even for most of our entire agricultural history humans had been trying to cultivate better and bigger plants and animals in the form of hybrid species. Most of our agriculture is based on selective breeding or artificial selection, plant grafting and so on. Sometimes creating new species can result in very aggressive new forms like the Africanized honey bee also known colloquially as "killer bee." There are some even more strange experimental hybrids that most people probably never heard of like zebroid (any equine + zebra), liger (female tiger + lion), narluga (beluga + narwhal), leopon (male leopard + female lion), geep (sheep + goat), or cama (lama + camel).

Why is all of this important? It is primarily significant for our understanding of what we are, and understanding of our physiology. When we understand that our body on the basic level is the same body that our hominin ancestors had, then we can try to understand what is our natural human way of life and diet. We need to have a diet that is congruent with the last hundreds of thousands of years of hominin evolution and even tens of millions of years. Difference between our modern way of life and way of life of our hominin ancestors (or in other words, we have their body, but we do not have their diet and lifestyle anymore) creates most of our imbalances in the form of chronic diseases and impaired quality of life. Our brain might evolve more than hominin brain, but our liver and internal organs, endocrine and immune system and our basic level of physiology did not. That is the key. Even our brain has the same neurons just a little more of them. This is the reason why we use animal testing experiments involving non-human primates for experimental research. Evolution works in tens of millions of years, not in tens of thousands. Abrupt lifestyle and diet changes caused by agricultural and industrial revolutions and by developing technologies cannot be matched by changes at the same speed and level in our biology. We have a form of lifestyle today that is not in balance with our own nature.

Take for example the trendy paleo diet. Paleo period ran from roughly 2.6 million to 10,000 years ago. Practitioners of this type of diet are trying to simulate the conditions of living in Stone Age hunter-gatherer conditions. They are trying to eat the diet that is in line with pseudo-hunter-gatherer lifestyle and give up the modern agricultural inventions like dairy, agrarian products, and processed foods. Now let stop here. Before we move on, we must understand the difference between hunter-gathering and foraging. These are two completely different diets. In order to be a hunter, we will have to be able to hunt as same as wild cats do. Because we are not adapted for chasing the prey, and an average human will not be able to chase down a single squirrel, we will have to depend on some technology. If we do not have the technology, then we depend on food that we can forage, and at the same time, we are the pray. Logically any form of hunting that will provide consistent food supply before developing of spears or traps will not be sustainable. So what was the real hominin diet and how such a diet might have influenced anatomy over time? Scientists can study the biochemical composition of fossil dental enamel. The biochemical composition can categorize the food in different types. These are cutting-edge scientific tests, and they indicate that before about 4 million years ago, hominids in Africa were eating a mostly vegan diet. It was a chimpanzee style diet based on fruits and some leaves. Even though the grasses and sedges were widespread and accessible in that period, the hominids appear to have neglected them for an extended time.

Most of our physiology was formed on this type of diet. It was just fruits and some leaves for us for tens of millions of years. A big "game changer" occurred about 3.5 million years ago when some members added grasses or sedges to their menus. It was a significant change. Later, we can see more differentiation. hominins from the genus Homo that evolved from Australopithecines like the 3-million-year-old fossil Lucy that is considered to be direct ancestor species of modern humans were increasing their food choices.

On the other hand, hominid known as Paranthropus boisei that existed side by side with them in eastern Africa was converging to a more specific diet. Scientists had initially nicknamed P. boisei the "Nutcracker Man" because of its large, flat teeth and powerful jaws. The recent analyses, on the other hand, have shown that it might have used its back teeth to grind grasses. As hominins got more prominent, in the same time consumption of grasses and sedges increased with bigger and stronger jaws and teeth's. Moreover, then the separation between Homo and Paranthropus happened. It looks probable that Paranthropus had a somewhat restricted diet, while members of the genus Homo were eating a wider variety of things. Because of this, the Paranthropus had a hard time adapting to changes in habitat and went extinct around one million years ago.

On the other hand, branch Homo that includes us did not. The arrival of the genus Homo was conventionally taken to coincide with the first use of stone tools. Next shift happened around a million years after first. Researchers have found, that hominins around 2.6 million years ago were beginning to eat the meat and bone marrow of antelopes. Were these antelopes hunted or scavenged is vigorously debated. At that period, our ancestors were eating a range of products from plants. I do not mean just fruits and young leaves, but also some of the natural leaves, and bark, invertebrate, and vertebrate animals, sages underground storage organs (such as tubers) to sedges. So the diet diversified little more but the information that we do not have is importance of every individual food in the overall diet. Since all of these foods are also consumed at least sporadically by all living monkeys of today including apes, these findings do not clarify what differentiate hominids apart from other primates. In other words, the diet was still somewhat similar to the diet of today living primates.

To reconstruct a more complex diet of later hominins, we must look to specific conditions in which they are evolving and then use the rules that would apply to that condition and behavior. Ecologists have been assembling these rules in an area of research called optimal foraging theory (OFT). OFT uses calculated models to predict how certain animals would forage in a different rage of given circumstances. OFT model estimates which foods should be eaten first and which ones would be passed over. One prediction, the golden rule if you like of foraging is that when high-quality foods are abundant, an animal will specialize in eating them disregarding other not so readily available lower quality options. In another case scenario when resources are scarce, an animal would broaden its diet in order to survive. In one study, different amounts of almonds were buried in view of chimpanzees. Some were still in the shell, and some were not. When they wanted to recover the nuts, chimpanzees firstly recovered those physically closer to them which means they had to spend less energy to get them (less pursuit time). They preferred bigger nuts then the smaller ones. Then they preferred those without shells (less processing time). Only at the end, the more distant, smaller, or with-shell nuts were picked up. This advocates the theory that at least some of the more intelligent animals like chimpanzees can remember optimal foraging strategies. In all of the studies that had been done on the OFT models the same conclusion can be made.

Moreover, all of them verify original estimates from OFT. The overall rate of addition of each food type to the diet will depend on the rarity of that food type in specific habitats, at particular seasons of the year. That statement is crucial to our entire discussion. Evidence suggests that our ancestors, and even we as modern humans, are omnivorous to some extent. We can adapt to the different environments to survive. Hominids did not spread across Africa, and then the entire globe, by utilizing just one foraging strategy. We did it by being flexible. However, again the percentage contribution of each food type to the diet will depend on the scarcity value of specific foods in specific habitats, at specific times of the year. Most crucial value for understanding is the percentage of the influx of different food types like meat for example in the overall diet. That will have an impact on the physiology of the species. The percentage is everything. What I mean would be explained in next chapters.

Evolutionary adaptation

"Whatever the life form, evolution selects for economy of resources" - Gregory Benford

An evolutionary adaptation is any heritable phenotypic character whose frequency of appearance in a population is the result of increased reproductive success. Adaptation is the development that the organism goes through in order to become accustomed to an environment. It is linked to evolution because it is a long process. One that occurs over many generations. Genetic change is what occurs. Some mutations may create genetic variation that will lead to differing characteristics of offspring and hence encourage adaptation. The genetic change that is the result of successful adaptation will always be beneficial to an organism. The more adapted species will have higher chances of survival, thus relating it to the process of natural selection.

Habitats do often change. Consequently, the process of adaptation is never finally complete. With time, it may result that the habitat changes to some extent and that species adapt to fit its surroundings better and better. For example, before snakes slithered, they had regular limbs. They were similar to lizards. In order to fit into small holes in the ground in which they could hide from predators, they lost their legs. Some of the modern snake species like boas and pythons still have a small stub in a place where their limbs used to be millions of years ago. It may also happen that the environment changes very little and that species do not need to adapt at all. Examples of this can be seen in so-called living fossils like jelly fish that evolved 550 million years ago or nautilus marine mollusks that remained largely unchanged for 500 million years. Biologists say that oldest living animals in the world today are ctenophores first emerged 700 million years ago. Also variations in the habitat may happen almost immediately, resulting in species to grow less and less well adapted and eventually to go extinct. To some extent, the adaptation influences every species in a particular environment even if that environment does not change. Van Valen theory was that even in a sound environment, competing species had to fight each other and continually evolve to maintain their relative standing. It is the so-called Red Queen's hypothesis.

What evolutionary adaptation have to do with our diet and why is this important? We have to understand how abrupt shifts in our environment caused by technological progress in our modern way of living can affect our biology that is not adapted to it and how it might affect our health. Other solution would be to act impulsively, emotionally and instinctively like most other animals. That is precisely what we can see when we visit hospitals and give most of our income on good service of modern medicine. Animals eat impulsively because they are conditioned to do it for survival. For all life on the planet Earth, food is not a choice. The hardest thing for an animal in the wilderness is to gain weight. The hardest thing for us is to lose it. If we start to treat food as a source of gratification and make dietary choices that are based on feelings and satisfaction, like it or not it will have health consequences. We have to find what type of diet is most congruent with our physiology and we have to look at our evolutional biology. If lifestyle and dietary choices are not congruent, our bodies will have a hard time adapting to it. Although we might still survive, we will have some level of maladaptation in the form of impaired quality of live, chronic disease and health issues.

For most of our evolution, we were slim in the state of constant hunger and constant physical activity, naked and were eating mostly vegan food. This was the case for all of our ancestor species and that means the time period of 50 million years. Obesity epidemic today is just maladaptation, and we will understand why by the end of this chapter. To better understand this thesis let us look at changes that happened in our modern history. When I say modern, I mean last 10,000 years that we have a record of. First most apparent to everyone would be a lightening of the skin. It has been theorized that dark skin pigmentation was the original condition for the genus Homo, including Homo sapiens. The problem arose when Homo sapiens moved into areas of low UV radiation. Light skin pigmentation is nothing more than a coping mechanism of our bodies for constant vitamin D shortages. Vitamin D is essential vitamin with different functions, for instance, one of them is calcium development. On another hand, the light-skinned individuals who now go back to live near the equator are at an increased risk of folate depletion. Folate depletion is associated with numerous types of cancers, especially skin cancer, DNA damage, and congenital disabilities. Just by entering a plane to go to habitat that we are not adapted for and doing activities like sunbathing on the beach can cause risk of skin cancer. It would be a good idea to drink beet juice while you are on vacation. It has the highest level of folate from all other food sources and folate is not the same substance as folic acid. Supplements have folic acid, and plants have folate. When they tested folic acid on rats their livers were able to convert folic acid into folate without any problems but we are not rats, and our liver is only able to convert a maximum of 400mg a day, so go with the beets and one 400 mg tablet.

Now let us investigate changes in diet and skin pigmentation. Scientific research confirmed in different ancient European genome studies that the hunter-gatherers in Europe could not digest lactose in milk at 8000 years ago. The first Europeans that domesticated wild animals were also unable to consume milk. The settlers who came from the Near East about 7800 years ago also couldn't. The Yamnaya pastoralists who came to Europe from the eastern steppes around 4800 years ago also couldn't. It was not until about 2300 BC about 4300 years ago, in the early Bronze Age, that lactose tolerance swept through Europe! When we look at today's world most of the population still can't digest milk. If lactose intolerant individuals consume lactose-containing products, they may experience bloating, nausea, abdominal pain, flatulence, and diarrhea. Lactose is split down to a regular usable sugar by specific enzyme called lactase created by cells in the wall lining of the small intestine. Production of lactase is turned off in mammals in adulthood because mammals breastfeed only in first periods after birth. Later in life in average conditions, it is not necessary to have this enzyme because no mammal will ever breastfeed again, except humans. Grown mammalian species do not breastfeed, and the organism is adapted to turn enzymes off to save energy. By domesticating wild animals and milking them, early farmers changed the condition of their habitat and in time organism adapted. Today only descendants of the European farmers can still digest milk. Black Africans cannot. Asians cannot. The statistic for lactose intolerance is like this. Approximately 65 percent of the entire human population has a reduced ability to digest lactose after infancy.

In comparison, 5 percent of people of Northern European descent are lactose intolerant. Had you ever seen African American celebrity in got milk commercial? Don't misunderstand me; there is, however, a lot of substances in milk that we cannot tolerate. Even if we are from dairy queen countries we still can't cope very well with things like cholesterol, a form of lacto morphine called casomorphin and estradiol (dairy consumption account for 60 to 80 percent of all estrogen consumed in the typical American diet). Opiates from mother's milk produce a sedative effect on the infant. That sedative effect is responsible for a good measure of the mother-infant bond. Milk has a drug-like effect on the baby (or other mammalian cubs), and it guarantees that the baby will bond with mom and proceed to nurse and get the nutrients. It is an evolutionary beneficial adaptation. Similar to heroin or codeine, casomorphins slow intestinal movements and have an antidiarrheal effect. The opiate effect is the reason why cheese can be constipating just as opiate painkillers are (in more detail it will be discussed in the chapter about milk in part 2 of the series).

When it comes to skin color, three separate genes produce light skin. European and also East Asian skin evolved to be much lighter only during the last 8000 years. First modern humans to initially settle Europe about 40,000 years ago are presumed to have had dark skin. Dark skin is beneficial in the sunny climate of Africa. Early hunter-gatherers around 8500 years ago, in Spain, and central Europe also had darker skin. Only in the far north where there are low light levels the environment will favor pale skin. When we look in the fossil record, then there is a different picture in hunter-gatherers in the far north. When examined all of the seven people from the 7700-year-old Motala archaeological site in southern Sweden, all had light skin gene variants. They also had a specific gene, HERC2/OCA2, which is responsible for blond hair, pale skin, and blue eyes. Around 8000 years ago in the far north ancient hunter-gatherers were pale and blue-eyed, but still, all of those people living in central and southern Europe still had darker skin. It was only after the first farmers from the Near East arrived in Europe that situation changed. They carried genes for light skin. As they have been interbreeding and mixing with the indigenous dark-skinned hunter-gatherers, one of their light-skin genes swept through Europe presumably because of the favorable environmental conditions that lack the sunny climate of Africa. It was only around 8000 years ago that people from central and south parts of Europe started to have lighter skin. Lack of sun, especially during winter, forced the adaptation and so natural selection has favored genetic adaptations to that problem by the paling of the skin that absorbs UV more efficiently.

The second line in adaptations to colder climates was favoring lactose tolerance. Vitamin D can be naturally found in some amount in regular milk. Vitamin D is not a vitamin. It is prohormone, a steroid with a hormone-like activity that regulates about 3% of the human genome from calcium metabolism, muscular function, immune system regulation and so on. The current medical knowledge associates vitamin D deficiency with contributing to the development of seventeen different autoimmune diseases, periodontal disease, cancers, congenital disabilities, stroke, and heart disease. Vitamin D insufficiency and in worse case even deficiency is a problem that has spread to the global level now. And why? Because we changed our habitat and started to wear clothes. If you are a Muslim woman in Sharia law country, it does not matter if you live in a sunny climate. If you are a black African and you start to live the modern way of life, meaning spending most of your time indoors, and in cars wearing t-shirts and pans you will be vitamin D deficient. Despite substantial daily sunlight availability in Africa and the Middle East, people living in these regions are often vitamin D insufficient or deficient ranging from 5% to 80%. Vitamin D insufficiency is rampant among African Americans. Even young, healthy blacks do not achieve optimal concentrations at any time of the year.

White people are more adapt to the northern climate. Black people are more adapt to the southern latitudes. Well at least before the Modern Era. Now we are not adapted to any climate. Why? Because we do not run naked not even during the summer, so we do not get any vitamin D for most of the year. We live indoors. Even being naked and exposed to the sunlight during summer was not enough for the northern geographical latitudes to sustain adequate vitamin D levels for entire year around. Our physiology adapted by paling our skin. Modern technology driven condition are 10-times worst. In the future, there will be no more Europeans, Africans, Hispanics, Indians, Hindus and so on. We will be physically similar and probably we will all have albinism as a result of adaptation if nothing is changed.

Groups of the Neanderthals were pale too. Some of them had more pigment, some less, some were pale and had red hear. If you do not believe this, we will go scientific. There is the receptor that activates melanin, the pigment that gives skin, hair, and eyes their color. It is known as melanin-activating peptide receptor melanocortin 1 (MC1R). It is present on the surface of melanocytes (cells that produce melanin). Melanocytes can make two different types of melanin. One is called eumelanin, and the other is pheomelanin. MC1R is a receptor that will decide which pigment will be produced. It acts as a switch. It will decide will it be red-and-yellow pigment pheomelanin or black-and-brown pigment eumelanin. In one genetic study, the scientific team led by Holger Römpler of Harvard University extracted, and sequenced MC1R gene from the bones of a 43,000-year-old Neanderthal from El Sidrón, Spain, and a 50,000-year-old one from Monti Lessini, Italy. The two Neanderthal samples both showed a point mutation that is not present in modern humans. If such a mutation is induced in human cells, it will cause an impaired MC1R activity. The mutation would cause red hair and pale skin in modern humans. To make sure that the MC1R gene mutation was not due to contamination of the sample from modern humans, the scientists tested around 4,000 people. None of the people tested had it. This genetic study showed that both Homo sapiens and Neanderthal had reached the same genetic adaptation by two different evolutionary pathways. Anthropologists had predicted a long time ago that do to the environment Neanderthals might have evolved to have pale skin. Work by Römpler and colleagues offers the first scientific evidence to support this thesis. So it is not that we inherited the blond gene from Neanderthals it is that evolution works similarly in similar conditions. When Neanderthals went into northern climates adaptation did the rest. Now when we have the modern technology, indoor lifestyle and all of the rest of the fancy new changes in the habitat that are not congruent with our physiology, the health problems will occur as a consequence of maladaptation. What experimental science have to say on how much vitamin D is adequate for the optimal health and in what form should we take it to balance back I will analyze in one of the chapters in book 3 of the series.

Another example would be exercise. We all know that training or exercise of any sort is healthy for us. We all had physical activity in schools. We have a different kinds of sports. We have soccer and basketball professional leagues for watching in leisure time, even Olympic Games. We glorify professional athletes as role models for our children and so on. Even our dog gets agitated if he does not receive his daily dose of walking. By why? Well, it is not because exercise itself is healthy. It is a stressful, painful experience full of sweat and the possibility of injuries that increases oxidative stress and leads to the creation of free radical DNA damage. Well if free radicals damage DNA and exercise leads to the creation of free radicals then how can it be that physical activity can be healthy? It is because our hominin ancestors lived by foraging. Physical activity was an essential component of their survival. You do not forage, you do not find food, you die. It is that simple. Also, the only reason exercise is healthy is because in a million years of evolution our body adapted to it. Our body expects it as a regular part of everyday life. When we do not exercise we are out of balance with our physiology, and when we do, we give our body's what they are expecting. When we go to the gym or do any other exercise like running on the treadmill, what we are actually doing is that we are simulating the conditions in the habitat of our hominin ancestors. When we look for scientific research about exercise, what will we find? Does exercise matter or it is just something to help us lose weight more rapidly? What we find is that individuals with low levels of physical activity are at higher risk of many different kinds of diseases like, heart disease, cancer, Alzheimer's disease and also early death by any cause. Long before that, inactivity increase lower-back pain, worsen arthritis symptoms and lead to anxiety. Exercise can help with lowering the risk of early death, high blood pressure, stroke, coronary heart disease, adverse blood lipid profile, type 2 diabetes, metabolic syndrome, colon cancer, breast cancer, depression, and can increase cognitive and mental health, sleep quality, immune system function and longevity. The Department of Health and Human Services (HHS) monitors this kind of research and releases periodically its Physical Activity Guidelines for Americans. Recommendations are that: "Adults between the ages of 18 and 64 exercise moderately (walking) for at least two hours and 30 minutes or vigorously (running, swimming, or cycling ten mph or faster) for at least an hour and 15 minutes weekly". That is about 11 minutes of running a day on the treadmill. For people who do not understand how to read this kind of releases, the keyword is for at least. The more is better. They are recommending what they think may be achievable. When we look at their charts of correlation between exercise and premature death all we can see is just a steady linear drop.

The Risk of Dying Prematurely Declines as People Become Physically Active

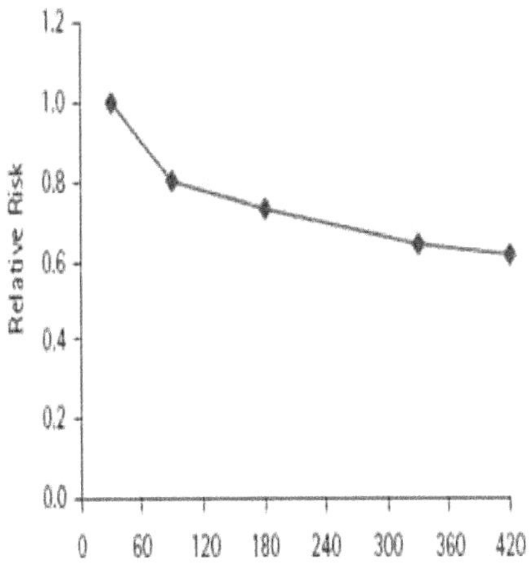

If we exercise 180 minutes a week, we will have 27% lower risk but if we exercise 420 minutes a week will have 38.5% lower risk, and this kind of correlation is found in all studies and systematic reviews and meta-analysis of cohort studies. In one study (Non-vigorous physical activity and all-cause mortality: systematic review and meta-analysis of cohort studies doi: 10.1093/ije/dyq104) they reviewed 22 studies that met inclusion criteria. Study containing 977,925 individuals (334,738 men and 643,187 women) and they found that 2.5h/week (equivalent to 30min daily for 5 days a week) compared with no activity was correlated with a decrease in mortality risk of 19%, while 7h/week of moderate activity compared with no activity reduced the mortality risk by 24%. The conclusion was that: "Being physically active reduces the risk of all-cause mortality." Going from no activity to the small amount was found to provide the most significant amount of benefit. However, that does not mean that if we are active that there is no additional benefit. Even at high levels of activity benefits still, accrue from the additional activity. The more and the longer the exercise, the more the benefits. No one will dispute this, and it is based on decades of scientific research.

So exercise by itself is correlated with the increase in DNA damage but it is healthy? How can that be? Again it is because of evolutionary adaptations in our biology. Our body expects it as a normal part of life and has adapted to it. When we exercise, the heart starts to contracts forcefully and frequently. That will increase blood flow through the arteries and allow our muscles to use more oxygen. Increase in blood flow will cause subtle changes in the autonomic nervous system, which controls the contraction and relaxation of these vessels. This adaptation leads to lowering blood pressure, more variable heart rate meaning ability of the heart to slow down or increase contractions when needed, lower resting heart rate overall which means increased efficacy of cardiovascular system with fewer beats to pump blood through the body, all aspects that have an impact in lowering cardiovascular disease. Exercise also lowers inflammation associated with the cardiovascular system. Exercise in research was able to cause around 30 percent dip in C-reactive protein levels, a marker of inflammation. Thirty percent drop is about the same drop that statin (the cholesterol drug) is able to cause. It beefs up the body's immune system and wards off cancer and other diseases. Exercise will help to maintain the bone mass and will reduce the risk of osteoporosis. Bones become stronger when forced to adapt to bear more weight than usual. When someone runs, muscle contractions will increase production of adenosine monophosphate-activated protein kinase (AMPK). This is an enzyme that promotes the breakdown of the fats that can interfere with the cells glucose transporters. AMPK can help in preventing type 2 diabetes. Research in rats shows that physical exercise boosts BDNF (brain-derived neurotrophic factor). BDNF is an essential factor in learning and memory. BDNF helps rats to remember how to navigate their way through mazes, and similar activity can be assumed in humans. Now the majority of people when they think about exercise they think about weight loss, and they think about weight loss because of the sex appeal. In cases of morbid obesity when the doctor tells patients to lose weight or die health considerations come into play. One hour of running depending on our weight will burn for example 520 calories at five mph for a 135-pound person. A man who weighs 175 pounds, nevertheless will burn 680 calories during a run of the same speed and duration. Can we run at 5mph every day for one hour? Mc Donald's large French fries will give us 461 calories and one large strawberry milkshake 458. We use our fat storage very well.

There is a way to stop oxidative free radical DNA damage if we eat an antioxidant-rich meal before the exercise. In this study (Acute and chronic watercress supplementation attenuates exercise-induced peripheral mononuclear cell DNA damage and lipid peroxidation; doi: 10.1017/S0007114512000992.) they wanted to see does eating antioxidant-rich food as watercress can help. They had given watercress to the subjects because watercress contains an array of nutritional compounds such as ß-carotene and α-tocopherol which may increase protection against exercise-induced oxidative stress. They just ate in acute (consumption two hours before exercise) and chronic (8-weeks consumption) period and then measured the effects. The main results show an exercise-induced rise in DNA damage and lipid peroxidation. Watercress reduced DNA damage and lipid peroxidation and decreased H2O2 accumulation following exhaustive exercise. These findings suggest that watercress ingestion has potential antioxidant effects against exercise-induced DNA damage. Also, we do not have to eat watercress, we have to eat any antioxidant-rich food in general. Food is more important than exercise as a general rule. Exercise is good, but it is not all junk you can eat then go and exercise kind of a deal. Physical activity is healthy, but without healthy nutritious antioxidant-rich diet, it cannot do miracles. Also, no we cannot just take a pill.

An evolutionary adaptation is not just adaptation to sun exposure, lactose tolerance or physical activity. Any lifestyle changes, every little thing that is not in line with evolutionary biology could potentially have health implications. Even the standard three meals a day plus snacks routine are not congruent with human evolution. Many nutritional experts will argue that we do not want to have oscillations in our blood sugar. The truth is that hypoglycemia is not good for the brain. Hypoglycemia was long considered to kill brain cells by depriving them of glucose every time we have it (Hypoglycemic brain damage. Metab Brain Dis. 2004 Dec;19(3-4):169-75). The truth is also that we cannot have hypoglycemia even if we want to if we do not have diabetes. An individual without signs of diabetes can stay within a relatively narrow band of blood sugar levels, ranging from about 70 to 130 mg/dl. The person with type 1 diabetes, oscillates widely between low and high levels depending on food intake. Type 2 profile is generally in a range much higher than that of a person with no diabetes. For a person without diabetes feeling of hunger is just that feeling of hunger and nothing more. There will be no harm to the brain. If you cannot deal with hunger and you have symptoms of hypoglycemia when you are hungry, you might have the first symptoms of prediabetes. Hypoglycemia symptoms include shakiness, fatigue, extreme hunger, irregular heart rhythm, and anxiety. If you do not have diabetes and you have skipped a meal you should not feel any of this only feeling of regular hunger.

The feeling of constant fullness, on the other hand, is not natural, and it is another example of maladaptation. Homo erectus did not have a fridge to go to in the middle of the night when he felt like eating. Hunger is a normal feeling for every animal. The only reasonable assumption is that hominins eat like any other animal when they found food in cycles of eating and hunger. Even when they are on a diet people will like to have a feeling of fullness. So here comes caffeine, hunger suppressors of different kinds and so on. If we can just find magical, all you can eat, weight loss diet. Hunger like exercise is something that our physiology is adapted to and expects it.

So what happens when we fast? First of all, fasting is not the same as starving. We only go to the starving mode when you do not have lipid tissue anymore. Before that, the body uses fat as energy. When we run out of fat storage, normal tissues became the food source, sort of speaking. However, not at the same rate. Muscle mass is metabolized first and only then the vital organs. We will not die or kill our brain or have any bad reaction if we go hungry. To be more precise starving mode comes when our fat deposits reach a level of essential fat. There are different types of body fat. They are not all the same. For instance, there is storage body fat that we all know about, but there is also essential body fat that many people have never heard about. Essential body fat is crucial for maintaining life and reproductive roles. The percentage of essential fat is 3–5% in men, and 10–13% in women. The demands for childbearing and other hormonal functions in woman makes essential body fat percentage little higher than that of a man. If we go below that level, we starve our organism. The body fat percentage (BFP) measures the total fat that you have. Body mass index measures total mass depending on tallness and are different from Body fat percentage. If we have greater muscle mass or larger bones, we will have higher BMI, so it tells us nothing about fat percentage. BMI is an only useful indicator for large groups of people, for example as a measurement on a population scale to tell us about overall obesity in population but is not a useful tool for determining the health status of an individual. BMI is a helpful pointer of overall health for a broad group of people because they do not exercise and have low muscle mass but BMI for itself tells us nothing. For example, there is so-called "skinny fat" body type, where you have high BMI and high BFP or in another words, you are obese and in the same time you have low muscle mass. Or you can have high BMI and low BFP like bodybuilders do. Body fat percentage in the leanest athletes is typically at levels of about 6–13% for men or 14–20% for women, this means full six pack abs and general shredded look. Also, there is something called visceral fat, and that is fat that we cannot see. The fat we may be capable of touching on our arms and legs is subcutaneous fat. This internal visceral fat encloses essential organs like the liver, heart, and kidneys and is called organ fat, intra-abdominal fat or visceral fat. When you are overweight you have more fat inside then you might think. A growing belly can be the result of both types of fat.

Carrying a large quantity of visceral fat is associated with stroke, heart disease, insulin resistance, osteoarthritis, gout, sleep apnea, asthma, breast cancer, and colorectal cancer. Individuals with a body mass index (BMI) of 30 or higher are considered obese. The term obesity is used to describe individuals who have a weight that can start to cause them health problems and is significantly above his or her ideal healthy weight. The term morbid obesity is used for individuals that have problems in their regular daily activities due to the excessive weight gain. It is a form of disability. Nearly 70% of American adults are either overweight or obese.

Moreover, there is the cherry on top called fatty liver, and I do not mean foie gras. Obesity is associated with a spectrum of liver abnormalities, known as nonalcoholic fatty liver disease (NAFLD). Most NAFLD patients are asymptomatic on clinical presentation, even though some may present a fatigue, dyspepsia and dull pain, a general feeling of being unwell and vague discomfort. Treatment for NAFLD involves weight reduction through lifestyle modifications, anti-obesity medication, and bariatric surgery. It is estimated that 75% of obese individuals are at risk of developing a simple fatty liver. The simple fatty liver is far from "simple" condition. Up to 23% of obese individuals are at risk of developing fatty liver with inflammation. Almost 10% of children may have NAFLD, due in large part to an alarming increase in childhood obesity. In morbidly obese individuals number is 95%. We can see the same thing in animals. Foie gras (French for "fat liver") is made of the liver of a duck or goose that has been forcefully and purposely fattened. It is a luxury food product trendy in France. Birds are fattened by force-feeding. The corn is forced down their throats with a feeding tube. The process is also known as gavage. Excessive feeding causes the birds to become obese. They have difficulty standing and their livers swell up to 10 times their average size. The same thing we can see in morbid obesity cases in humans. It is animal cruelty to the extreme. It is a painful condition with engorged livers that distend their abdomens. Because of the pain, the birds are usually very aggressive. They may attack each other out of stress and rip out their own feathers. The technique of gavage dates as far back as 2500 BC. The ancient Egyptians did utilize this technique first before it spread to other countries.

Why so many people lose control over eating and force feed themselves? Because of modern technology, or in other words because they can. There is a hormone called leptin the satiety hormone, made by fat cells. The fatter we are, the more hormone in the blood. Leptin the satiety hormone, is opposed by the actions of the hormone named ghrelin, the hunger hormone. Both hormones act on the receptors in the brain to regulate appetite. The balance of these two hormones is necessary to achieve overall energy balance in the body. In obesity, a decreased sensitivity to leptin occurs. This is a big problem that will result in a brain inability to detect satiety despite high energy stores in the rest of the body.

Why does this happen? The basis for leptin resistance in obese human subjects is unknown. If leptin levels remain persistently raised due to overeating, there may be downregulation of the leptin receptors and hence decreased sensitivity to the hormone. In humans, and actually in any other animal low leptin level induced by low calorie diet results in a decrease in plasma leptin concentration triggering high levels of constant hunger. This may explain the high failure rate of dieting. Low leptin levels are likely to be a powerful stimulus to weight gain.

On the other hand, anorexia nervosa patients also have deficient leptin levels but with one big difference. When they refeed themselves, their plasma leptin concentration will increase rapidly and reach roughly normal levels long before normal weight is achieved. Thus keeping them anorexic. Excessive leptin production and its effect on the feeling of fullness could play a permissive role in the pathogenesis of this condition.

Where is the malfunction? Obesity dilemma and epidemic remain shrouded in complexity and mystery. There is a thesis, and this is my personal opinion also that obesity conditions are `mal-adaptations' of actual current modern lifestyle to our genome (Fernandez-Real & Ricart 1999). In other words, maladaptation is something that occurs in abrupt shift of habitat that physiology is not adapted to cope with. There is no underlining difference between a low level of leptin activation in the brain that leads to overeating and low levels of something else for example serotonin activation in the brain that leads to symptoms of clinical depression. Low levels of "something" means that "something" else is off. In the case of obesity, the standard regulatory system will tell the brain that we have fat deposits stored for an extended period and that we can endure little hunger. Overeating in my way of looking at things is a form of drug addiction. Like I wrote before Homo erectus did not have a fridge to go to in the middle of the night when he felt like eating. Hunger is a normal feeling for every animal. Hominins eat like any other animal when they find food in cycles of eating and hunger. They could never become fat due to scarcity, so they never developed adaptation to the abundance of food. Our mind still thinks that if we do not eat all that we can we will starve to death in the upcoming drought. Even our concept of beauty changed. I do not mean what we were thinking is pretty in ancient Egypt or Persia. That is a form of modern agricultural civilization with societal structures. Let's look at some Stone Age Venus figurines.

1. Venus of Gagarino, Russia 20,000 BC; 2. Figurine féminine dite manche de poignard de Brassempouy, 23,000 BC; 3. Venus de Losange Italy 25,000 BC; 4. Venus of Tepe Sarab Iran 6500 BC; 5. Neolithic Hassuna Princess „Idol," 6500-5700 BC Mesopotamia; 6. Malta Venus 4500 BC; 7. Venus of Willendorf Austria 24000 BC; 8. Venus of Moravany Slovakia 23000 BC; 9. Ceramic Figurine of a Woman 5300 BC, The British Museum; 10. Venus from Hohle Fels, Germany 38,000 BC; 11. Cave Ghar Dalam, Malta 5400 BC; 12. Catalhohuk 6000 BC; 13. Venus of Monruz 10,000 BC, Switzerland; 14. Venus

of Dolní Věstonice, Czech Republic 29,000 BC; 15. Venus of Anatolia, Turkey 6000 BC; 16. Inanna (Ishtar) Mother Goddess, Mesopotamia 2000 BC.

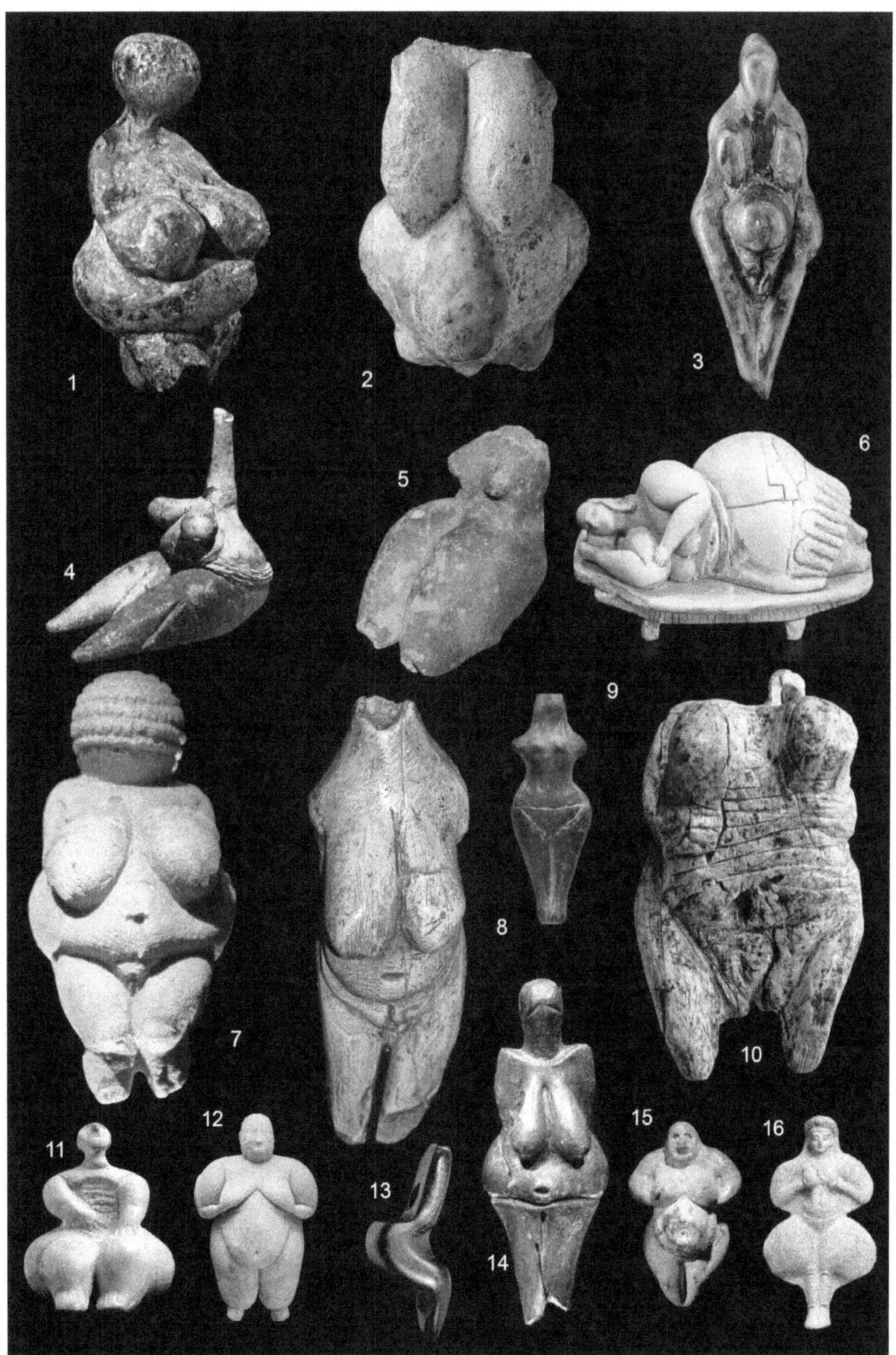

In contrast, hunter-gathers idealized morbid obesity. Difference between foraging and hunter-gathering and agriculture, and then agricultural societies and our modern industrial ones are significant. They are enormous regarding evolutionary biology. It was all about survival. The skinny, malnourished female was in danger if became pregnant. Just Iodine deficiency can cause congenital abnormalities, neurological cretinism, mental deficiency, spastic diplegia, cretinism and a long list of other things. Low zinc levels can cause fetal growth retardation and congenital abnormalities; calcium deficiency can lead to poor fetal skeletal development; low iron levels can cause fetal growth retardation. Maternal under-nutrition can produce a child with renal dysfunction, organ dysfunction of testes, ovaries, brain, heart, liver, small intestine and so on. Mothers today spend their entire pregnancy worrying about what to do to have a healthy baby. In Ice Age in Europe during winter (last glacial period from 110,000 – 11,700 years ago), a malnourished pregnant woman would have many problems. And no there were no contraceptive pills in that era. Morbid obesity is a symbol of fertility or a symbol of successful pregnancy and symbol of life itself. Our paleo grandparents did not understand the full range of functioning of biological principles, but they for sure understand the role of adipose tissue for survival. For more than hundred thousand years it was the way of life, ever since our ancestors moved out of Africa and entered colder climates, and even in Africa actually, there was no overabundance of sources of food around also. In snow and ice and caves with constant hunger and other hominins around competing for food, it was the worst case scenario. That is why we can see morbid obesity Venuses.

After the Neolithic Revolution, it all shifted rapidly. When we do not hunt and forage anymore and now grow our own food, we do not depend on habitat anymore. We make our own. It was the first significant change after control use of fire by Homo erectus, and later Homo sapiens use of spears and traps technologies. So habitat shifted. Overproduction of crops started. A number of people erupted. There were first larger cities and societal hierarchies, i.e., priests and kings and other important people. Also, just like in Egypt concept of fertility shifted everywhere. Goddesses became slimmer, stories grew into religion and morphed into the culture. Even inter-gender relations changed. Feminism is not a modern invention. For example, in ancient Egypt, the woman was regarded as entirely equal to men as far as the law was concerned. They had the right to own the property. They could own a private business and sign contracts. They could also become pharaohs on rare occasions. Life of regular people was much more similar to our own. In Egypt, during the New Kingdom, there was a substantial middle class. Their houses although lacking modern inventions like electricity would have been much the same size as houses of middle-class people of North America today. Houses of wealthy individuals were much more prominent. The wealthy home had many rooms beside the living room, the same as modern houses. There were bathrooms, storage rooms, bedrooms, office for the head of the house and so on. All of these commodities because of cultivating wild plants and domesticating animals and mud from the Nile. No need for fat goddess anymore. In other parts of the world pretty much the same. Ancient Egyptians were more closely related to Europeans than Africans. Acquiring genetic information from ancient mummies showed that ancient Egyptians are most closely related to Neolithic and Bronze Age samples in the Levant, as well as to Neolithic Anatolian and European samples, and cultures in all that area were similar (Ancient Egyptian mummy genomes suggest an increase of Sub-Saharan African ancestry in post Roman period Nature Communications 8, Article number:15694(2017) doi:10.1038/ncomms15694). Some were more patriarchal, some extremely, some less butt once the technology allowed the population to rise and there were big cities, things changed. The woman would be able to escape, and that is it. She will find some other men or become a prostitute or find another job if she can or if she had money problem solved.

In contrast in hunter-gatherer caves running off is not an option. Mansplaining was the law of the land. No police to call no firefighters. If a tribe of hunter-gatherers came back to cave escaping an angry pack of wild wolves eager to rip flash of their faces without finding any animal to catch or nothing to forage and found that one problematic wife had again eaten more then she had been entitled to do, she would be kicked out probably. In that kind of environment that means a death sentence. If she is lucky, she will find a group of other humans or Neanderthals, but that is unlikely too. Neanderthals too have females in the caves and they surely don't like to split food with some human stray. Other humans will not touch her either because when we see a lonely stray, we know what is going on. Nobody likes trouble. Even for males, it was the same. Kicking out of the tribe was a death sentence. No survival chances. That kind of conditioning in big city's collapses. Every man for himself. Homo homini lupus est. Technology at the end is what defines our relations. Woman gender should incorporate the April, 21 in their rites as a day of worship instead of the March the 8. God of technology did more to woman equality than any social-political movement ever did.

So what happens when we fast? Let us look what happens to the body when we go into fasting mode (not starving mode). First, the body will burn readily available calories in the form of stored sugar glycogen. Most sugar is stored primarily in the cells of the liver and the muscles, hydrated with water. So we will lose some water weight. If you do not know this, you can be surprised when you go on a diet and lose water and be happy, to gain it all back after. Water loss released from glycogen and sodium is usually the culprit for dramatic first-week weight loss. Sodium will be flushed out by urine with kidneys if sodium is not needed, but if there is excessively significant amount of sodium in our body for our kidneys to excrete, the sodium would not be able to leave the body and then it will start to accumulate causing us to hold water. If you want to flush out excess sodium, then replace the heavy salted processed foods with unsalted natural ones and increase your water intake. That will result in a sudden loss of weight, without any dieting or calorie restriction, but it will be mostly water. Just water, not fat. In the liver, glycogen reserves can build up to 5–6% of the organ's flesh weight (100–120 grams in an adult). Muscles have a much lower concentration of glycogen, in the range of one to two percent of the total muscle mass. The untrained individual holds typically about 400 grams of glycogen that is stored in the entire body, in both muscles and the liver. A trained professional athlete can hold double that amount. This amount of glycogen is enough to last for several hours of intensive exercise without replenishment. When we train our body adapts, and condition improves. Professional athletes also do something called carbohydrate loading after the exercises to force their body to adapt by increasing the storage capacity of intramuscular glycogen stores. There are some studies done on this. If we take caffeine or drink coffee glycogen stores tend to be replenished more rapidly. Long-distance athletes often experience glycogen depletion. It is called "hitting the wall". In professional sport, it has a powerful influence because after depleting sugar reserve, fatigue follows and sometimes to the point that it is difficult to move. This is the reason when you see athlete bonking. Bonking is not the state in which you are just feeling tired. Bonking is when your glycogen reserve stores get so low that your brain starts to run out of energy and then shuts your body down. The liver will begin to break down fat and protein to form energy immediately. The problem is that this process takes time and until gluconeogenesis kicks in, an athlete may experience symptoms of hypoglycemia. If this happens, it will not be uncommon to see professional athletes collapse from the extreme fatigue. Hypoglycemia comes with dizziness, blurred vision, hallucinations. Loss of consciousness may also occur under these conditions. The combined use of several different energy sources that allow extended high muscular power outputs that can be maintained for an extended period is big deal in professional sport and research. Also, no we cannot go on a diet before the marathon to tap to gluconeogenesis and then run. Running a marathon using fat alone as a fuel source is not plausible.

Moreover, our body can only process a limited amount of carbohydrates per hour, around 30-60 grams depending on individual efficiency. Now you probably won't race a marathon, but it is essential to understand how the body works if you want to exercise, you can potentially do yourself damage, or don't get the desired results. In bodybuilding it is a big deal also because taping into muscle mass for energy is not desired course. After glycogen depletion from 16 hours to 72 hours, the body will lean heavily on amino acids and protein catabolism for energy creation. Amino acids will be used, and some of the muscle mass will be lost when going on a fast with or without exercise. We can try to minimize it, but some amino acids will be used for energy. Loss of some of the tissue as we will see, has an evolutionary purpose and health benefits if done moderately. It is normal for all animals including humans, and because our bodies have adapted to expect it in same way as physical activity, it will have a negative impact on our health if we do not incorporate fasting in our regular life. After this initial period, our metabolism will shift to ketosis where it gets almost all of its energy from ketone bodies from fat metabolism. The basal metabolic rate will drop also, or in other words, the use of energy will become more efficient. We can last to a period of 2.5 to 3 months just drinking water depending on how much fat we have to begin with. If we have large amounts of fat, we can last much longer, but nutrient deficiencies will occur.

There is a study (Features of a successful therapeutic fast of 382 days duration, Postgrad Med J. 1973 Mar; 49(569): 203–209) where a 27-year-old male patient that was described as grossly obese fasted under supervision for 382 days. During the 382 days of his fast, he was given vitamin supplements daily. From day 93 to day 162, he was given potassium and from day 345 to day 355 only he was given 2.5 g of table salt daily. No other drug treatment was given. The patient lost 276 pounds during his 382 days of fasting (0.7 a day just on water alone, so don't believe in the magic diet plans that many are selling). This study suggests that the human body can adapt to total starvation for prolonged periods. As long as the body fat reserves exist and as long as the subject is supplemented with vitamins, minerals, and of course water there will be no serious health complications. Having three meals plus snacks is a modern invention. To recap some amino acids will be used and some of the tissue mass will be lost when we go on a fast with or without exercise, and the basal metabolic rate will drop also. This sound bad right. Well, our physiology is adapted to it and just like exercise it expects it. Hunger is a normal feeling for every animal. It might be contra-intuitive to think that losing regular tissue and slowing metabolism is a healthy thing.

We want to have muscle mass as much as possible and fast metabolism as much as we can so that we can eat more and don't gain weight but evolutionary biology will again tell us what is healthy. I am going to use a quote from the U.S. Department of Health & Human Services National Institute on Aging website: "Since the 1930s, investigators have consistently found that laboratory rats and mice live up to 40 percent longer than usual and also appear to be more resistant to age-related diseases when fed a diet that has at least 30 percent fewer calories than they would normally consume. Now researchers are exploring whether and how caloric restriction will affect aging in monkeys and other nonhuman primates." We have human studies now. The calorie restriction response exists in nearly all of the species tested to date, and probably had evolved very early in the history of life on Earth as a mechanism to increase the chances of surviving periodic shortages. There is the difference between fasting and prolong calorie restriction but the underlining mechanism is the same, and caloric restriction will prolong life expectancy much more than fasting periodically although even fasting periodically will have beneficial effects on longevity. The benefit comes from two main reasons. There are other benefits like improved insulin sensitivity, regulating inflammatory conditions in the body and starving off cancer cell formation, detoxifying, improving eating patterns, hormonal balancing. However, there is two main reason on a cellular level that underlines all of the other benefits that sprout out of these two.

Firstly, when we fast blood levels of insulin drop significantly, and blood levels of growth hormone may increase as much as 5-fold. Insulin and growth hormone play antagonistic roles against one another. When one is elevated, the other will be low. When we go to sleep we fast for 10 hours, insulin drops and HGH (human growth hormone) rises. When HGH rises we grow, especially if you are in puberty. HGH stimulates growth, cell reproduction, and cell regeneration. It is thus essential in human development. The reason why animals and humans sleep is to ensure the rise of HGH and regeneration. Since animals are particularly vulnerable while sleeping, evolutionary, there must be advantages that will outweigh this considerable disadvantage. Rats deprived of sleep die in a few weeks. Sleep-deprived rats lose weight despite increased food intake and progressively fail to regulate body temperature. They also develop infections, suggesting an impairment of the immune system. It is not just the brain that needs to regenerate and you cannot regenerate your body if insulin is pumping through the bloodstream. We need to sleep plus we need to fast from time to time just like animals in nature.

Secondly, when we fast our cells initiate important cellular repair processes and change in which genes they express. We start to regenerate and allow for cleansing and detoxification of the body. One of the reasons why sick people have a low appetite is that there are in the process of intensive regeneration. In medical terms that regeneration is called autophagy. In the ancient Greek word "phagy" means eating and the word "auto" meaning self, so autophagy means literary self-eating. You self-eat yourself every day. When any cell in our body dies, it will not go to waste. What happens is recycling. Autophagy is a completely natural physiological method in the body that deals with the destruction of cells. It controls homeostasis or regular functioning by protein degradation and destruction and turnover of the destroyed cell organelles for the new cell formation. During cellular stress (deprivation of nutrients) the process of autophagy is increased. Autophagy has the ability to likewise also destroys the cells under certain conditions. There is a form of programmed cell death (PCD) and there is autophagy induced cell death. Two different types. Programmed cell death is commonly termed apoptosis. Autophagy is termed as non-apoptotic programmed cell death with different pathways and mediators from apoptosis. Also, this is the key to calorie restriction and fasting. If the cell is precancerous for example or damaged or mutated in any way and doesn't want to "go" by apoptosis, autophagy cell death can help her "go". After glycogen depletion, we will go into increase autophagy, and our body will lean heavily on amino acids and protein catabolism for energy creation. Amino acids will be used, and some of the muscle mass will be lost.

Moreover, it is a good thing. Why? Because our organism is much smarter, then we think. Our heart is the muscle too, but it would not be touched. First goes glycogen, then fat, then muscle then vital organs, and then we die from malnutrition. It is a brilliant plan to sustain life throughout hunger. If there is a "bad" cell and "good" cell and some of the cells needs to "go" for energy, well first on the line is the bad cell. First on the line to get rid of are the parts of the system that might be damaged or old. The inefficient parts. The absence of autophagy is believed to be one of the main reasons for the accumulation of damaged cells, and this can lead to serious health complications. If we start severely damaged by chemotherapy or other toxins, fasting cycles can generate, literally, an entirely new immune system. Exercise by itself is able to increase autophagy in a situation where autophagy already happens. The more intensive the exercise is, the more effective it will be. However, if we eat and work out the exercise alone would not be beneficial. The fastest way to shut down autophagy is to eat high amounts of complete protein. What this will do is to stimulate IGF-1 (Insulin-like growth factor 1) and mTOR (rapamycin), which are potent inhibitors of autophagy. IGF-1 (Insulin Growth Factor) is somewhat responsible for muscle growth. However, IGF-1 catastrophic side effect is cancer. It is best to limit protein to about 50 to 70 grams per day, depending on lean body mass. When we ingest large amounts of protein, our liver detects it, and the response is:" Hey let's grow stuff, we have all essential amino acids now." It starts pumping IGF-1. In fasting state liver GH (growth hormone) binding is decreased, so more of the GH is left in the bloodstream. In protein restriction, GH receptors are maintained but not for IGF-1. When we have advanced to be a fully grown humans, cell growth is something we will like to maintain in the optimal level and not accelerate. There are studies to show that there is no correlation between IGF level and protein intake but these studies did not account for animal versus plant protein.

When we ingest an incomplete source of protein, meaning it lacks some of the essential amino acids, it will not signal the IGF-1 release. Plant protein seems to lower the levels of IGF-1. It is not just about the overall amount of protein consumed but also the source (Study reference: The Associations of Diet with Serum Insulin-like Growth Factor and Its Main Binding Proteins in 292 Women Meat-Eaters, Vegetarians, and Vegans - Cancer Epidemiol Biomarkers Prev. 2002 Nov;11(11):1441-8). It is because of the protein profile. Vegans for instance that eat 7 to 18 servings of soy meals a day may end up with circulating IGF-1 levels that is relative to those who eat meat. That is because soy has complete protein. Some other plants have high quality proteins too. High consumption level of protein in diet have other negative effects regardless. I will write about it more in the chapter about protein in second book of the series.

The good news is that we can use autophagy to clean our genetic base, the bad news is that we do not do it anymore. In past nature forced us by not providing enough resources. Today we eat regularly and even if we go hungry that will not last enough to deplete our glycogen stores. There is a form of diet that is not related to weight loss primarily. Even some bodybuilders appear to try it. It is diet primarily designed for utilizing autophagy called intermittent fasting. What they try to do is to limit the intake of calories by 4 to 8 hours a day. So the rest of the time there will be fasting to tap into this mode of healing. However, there will not cut on the calories they will be just consuming them in the restricted period. Some studies show that this too can have beneficial effects. There is truth in the statement that meal frequency is not nearly as important as the quantity and quality of food consumed. Thus logically if we still eat all of our calories on the period of 4 hours and are active rest of the time, it is still unlikely that we will burn all of our glycogen stores because we replenish them every day.

In that sense, intermitting fasting would not be able to tap into the same healing mechanism at the level of calorie restriction. If we eat less and go into calorie restriction, it does not matter because we will be in deficit no matter when we eat. It will be a good idea to put exercise on a regimen of intermittent fasting just before the end of the fast, to deplete the glycogen stores, or we can combine all three methods. Calorie restriction with intermittent fasting with physical activity. To go around this, there is Alternate day fasting (ADF). It involves a 24-hour fast followed by a 24-hour non-fasting period. Then there are whole-day fasting cycles that specify various ratios of fasting to non-fasting days, such as the 5:2 diet. You eat for five days, then fast on water or vegetable juices for two. So far studies done on animal models have shown that fasting improves indicators of health like blood pressure, insulin sensitivity, and inflammation. Intermittent fasting in my personal view started as a convenient way to do a calorie restriction diet. To do full calorie restriction diet is a hard choice. The most of the population will not do it. Intermitting fasting line is to go and fast 1 or 2 days a week and clean our cells, reset our metabolism take control of our hunger cravings and so on. That will help our body to go into autophagy and high HGH levels and will start healing mechanism. However, there is another essential benefit of calorie restriction, and that is lowering the basal metabolic rate. If we have a car with a million horsepower's, it will burn a gallon of fuel in a millisecond, but if we have a car that runs on one horsepower, it will go much longer. It is called efficiency. When you force yourself to become more efficient in burning of energy you go longer.

Calorie restriction is not calorie restriction our entire life. It is only restriction in the beginning period. Our physiology will adapt to hunger to some extent by becoming more efficient with calories that it has. Basal metabolic rate has the ability to slow down, but only to some extent. Your body will enter the starvation response and will go through physiological changes that reduce metabolism in response to a lacking of food. Human body have some level of ability to adapt and structure itself known as deprivation response (i.e., metabolic adaptation). There was a study done on eight individuals living in isolation in Biosphere 2. Biosphere 2 is an Earth Systems science research facility located in Oracle, Arizona. It was initially designed to determine the viability of closed ecological systems to support human life in outer space. First experiment was conducted on eight individuals for two years. After the experiment were finished, the metabolic rate of these eight isolated individuals was measured and compared with a control group that initially had similar physical characteristics. The starvation response managed to reduce the metabolic rate for 180 kcal on average in daily total energy expenditure. If you eat regularly 2000 calories and you start to restrict the calories your metabolism slows down to 1800 calories at average. Then when you came back to eat these 1800 calories, it is not restriction anymore. It is in a sense because you are at an artificially lowered metabolic rate so if you start overeating again your basal metabolic rate will go up, but if you stay in this level you will not starve and die. You can live in this new state. People have this kind of idea about calorie restriction diet that you are restricted continuously. In a sense, you are because you operate at a lower metabolic rate, but you are not in the physical sense or you will eventually die. And that is the reason why calorie restriction prolongs life. Slowing down metabolism meaning prolonging life through efficiency. Burning fuel means stress in the form of oxidative damage to the DNA that needs to be repaired. Can you gain a muscle on caloric restriction? Probably just some level of body recomposition. If you have some kilograms to loose then lowering by 400 calories can increase muscle and lower fat deposits at the same time if you do resistance training. But if you are already calorie restricted at the optimal level then no, your body has already lowered your metabolism as much as it can. There is calorie in calorie out equation based on the first law of thermodynamics. It might be possible on intermittent fasting cycles. Five days of resistance training than two days of aerobic training plus fasting.

One other thing. When we start building muscle our metabolism can slow down if we do not increase calories, it will adapt to some extent. We do not need to start overeating excessively just because we go to the gym. That will give you dirty bulk. One hundred grams of flesh have around 25 grams of protein and 150 calories, and you cannot grow at the rate of 100 grams of muscle mass a day. In my opinion, when we start resistance training, it would be wise to raise calorie consumption at the level of what is burned during the exercise plus a little more, at top 200 calories more than that. Raising it higher is excess that goes into adipose tissue, basically the waste of energy that has to be burned at some point. Overeating with the excuse:" I go to the gym", is not a good idea.

So what happens when our regular metabolism burns energy for life? Well, some of that energy escapes and do damage to DNA, and some of the damaged cells naturally end their life cycle and die. In their place comes new ones from the division. The higher the metabolism, the higher the damage, and the higher the division. Every time cell divide it clips telomere in half. A telomere is a small area of repeated nucleotide sequences at each end of a chromosome. The purpose of the telomere is to keep the end of the chromosome from deterioration or fusion with other neighboring chromosomes. During chromosome duplication, the enzymes that duplicate DNA can maintain their duplication unit at the end of a chromosome. What happens is that in each duplication, the end of the chromosome is shortened. After too many divisions telomeres are gone, and there are no more divisions only death. It is a process called aging. We can slow this process down by slowing oxidative damage with high levels of antioxidants in diet, and we can slow it down by increasing energy efficiency. The problem is that nothing in nature is 100% effective. Some of the oxygen in our cells escapes in the form of free radicals and do their oxidation elsewhere. Oxidative stress happens when an oxygen molecule splits into single atoms with unpaired electrons. These aggressive molecules are called free radicals. They are so aggressive that they will attack the nearest stable molecule trying to steal its electron particle. When the attacked particle is left with no electron, it will become the free radical itself. The process is going to create a chain reaction. Once the process is started, the final result is the disruption of a living cell. Free radicals are created as a part of normal metabolism.

Four different mechanisms produce endogenous (your body creates them) free radicals. Production of free radicals cannot be entirely stopped. It is surprisingly amusing to me that oxygen, an element indispensable for life is also responsible for our death. It is not plausible to directly measure the number of free radicals in the body. The more fuel we burn, the faster we burn out. Have you ever asked yourself how many heartbeats a common man has in their life? It turns out each animal gets around a billion beats. Smaller animals have higher metabolic rates, and their heart is beating faster. When we calculate the number of beats for different size of different species of animals the magic number is one billion. Horses, rabbits, cats, pigs, elephants, whales, it does not matter, it is always one billion. Other than small dogs. They got the short end of the stick. In contrast, humans and chickens are champions in that we get more than double of the usual natural number. Around 2.21 billion for us and 2.17 billion beats for chickens. The quicker your metabolism is the faster you will oxidase and die. It is called the rate of living theory. Max Rubner had first proposed the concept in 1908. He observed that larger animals always outlived smaller ones and that the larger animals had slower metabolisms. A further affirmation was given to these observations by the discovery of Max Kleiber's law in 1932. Kleiber assumed that basal metabolic rate could correctly be predicted by taking 3/4 the power of body weight. This theory is colloquially known as the mouse-to-elephant curve. Support for this theory has been reinforced by studies linking a lower basal metabolic rate (evident with a lowered heartbeat) to increased life expectancy. Grand Tortoise can live up to 150 years. Hummingbirds have the highest metabolism of any homoeothermic animal. Their hearts beat at over 1263 beats per minute. At night, they enter tupor, a form of deep sleep. In tupor their heart rate drops to 50 beats a minute to conserve energy. The average lifespan of a wild hummingbird is 3-10 years.

One species that stick out for longevity are Macaws. Birds in general average some 2 to 3 times the longevity of mammals. There are specific avian groups that are even longer-lived than this overall average. Why and how, nobody knows. The interesting fact is that oxygen consumption in a unit of time in bird cells can go as high as 2.5 times that of mammals. If we combine this fact of high metabolic rate and oxygen consumption with the long lives of birds, we have unsolved scientific phenomena. If we calculate the numbers, we can see that some long-lived avian cells may be able to live as much as 20 times longer than some of the short-lived mammals such as mice and five times that of regular long-lived mammals such as humans. If we find out how and what the secret is, we could possibly have five times of life expectancy. Birds have evolved some protection against free radical damage. They have evolved some effective mechanism for protection from the buildup of free radicals. The circumstances of those protective measures so far remain elusive. Studies within those sectors of oxidative free radical protection have so far been restricted, and the evidence has been moderately conflicting. It will be significant in pharmaceutics, it already is. Universal strong antioxidant and calorie restriction pill, all we can eat and still have the benefits. There is one substance called Compound SRT1720. SRT1720 mimics dietary restriction, lessening many of the harmful effects of the high-fat diet and obesity with no signs of toxicity even after 80 weeks of treatment. We cannot buy this stuff yet.

What we can have at present is something in the form of strong universal antioxidants like Astaxanthin or MegaHydrate, but more research had to be done, especially to see if the high rate of dietary antioxidants had an adverse effect on immune cells that use the release of oxygen free radicals like macrophages. There is also evidence that antioxidants like beta-carotene can harm us if not taken in a whole food way. In the future, there will probably be much more research done in this area. In one study that I will mention (Analysis of telomere length and telomerase activity in tree species of various lifespans, and with age in the bristlecone pine Pinus longaeva; Biogerontology. 2005;6(2):101-11) they analyzed one type of bristlecone pines, Pinus longaeva. It is the oldest known living eukaryotic organism, with the oldest on record turning 4780 years old in 2015. In this study, researchers did a detailed investigation of telomere length and telomerase activity. Telomerase is a ribonucleoprotein an enzyme that adds a species-dependent telomere repeat sequence to the end of telomeres. It lengthens the telomeres. Some cells, not all of them can maintain telomere length by the action of this enzyme, thus keeping themselves from death. The conclusions of the research confirm the assumption that: "Both increased telomere length and telomerase activity may directly/indirectly contribute to the increased life-span and longevity evident in long-lived pine trees (2000-5000 year life-spans)." In the future, we will have some t-pill maybe, but until that time we need to correct our lifestyle. Periodical fasting can be one way. It will help us as much as exercise and as much as a good diet.

However, who will actually do this? Ascetic monks. On a population scale, it is not sustainable and actually on a population scale we see reverse action. For us, it is all about how to overcome our metabolism and calorie adaptation so that we can eat more, lose weight more quickly and have six-pack abs and French fries at the same time. Many people describe dieting to be a 50% physiological battle and a 50% psychological battle, and they are not far off from the mark unless you can deal with the intensive food cravings you face. Most people on a diet are running a calorie deficit of around 500 calories below maintenance. After metabolic adaptation takes place, we can see how fast weight loss would go.

Moreover, just around the corner are birthday parties, holidays and of course cheat meals. Eating for pleasure is nothing new.

I wrote before that I think obesity is a form of drug addiction. I will explain now why. In nature, there is no free sugar or free fat. Energy is stored in complex whole food packages and one or the other form. Nuts and seeds have their energy stored in the form of fat and grains for example in the form of complex sugars or carbohydrates, and they come with fiber and other substances. Our brain had never been exposed to refined sugar or fat before and especially never been exposed to a combination of the two in high doses all at once. For example, when we eat ice-cream or milk chocolate, we have sugar and fat combination that does not exist in nature. What happens in the brain is the same thing that happens when you inhale crack cocaine. Crack cocaine itself is a refined product. Cocaine naturally occurs only in coca plant. You cannot get high at that high level if you chew the leaves as Indian tribes do. It is a traditional stimulant to overcome hunger, fatigue, and thirst. It is considered predominantly effective against altitude sickness. In folk medicine, coca leaves are also used as an anesthetic and to alleviate the pain of a headache, rheumatism, wounds, etc. Before stronger modern anesthetics were available, it also was used for childbirth, wounds and broken bones. Because coca constricts blood vessels, it is also used to oppose bleeding. Some other conditions that indigenous people had used coca are for treatment of malaria, asthma, ulcers, diarrhea and other digestive problems. It is also thought that it has aphrodisiac qualities and that also improves longevity. Modern studies have supported a number of these medical applications. However, when we extract or in other word refine the cocaine or sugar or fat it is a different story. We can eat poppy seeds as much as we like but when we refine the opium and inject it into the vein or drink the poppy tea, well, here comes the magic dragon. In typical research involved with hunger and weight regulation the focus was on so-called metabolic or homeostatic hunger. Metabolic hunger is driven by real physiological necessity and is most commonly identified with the rumblings of an empty stomach. By the 1980s researchers had mapped out all of the main hormones and neural connections responsible for metabolic hunger.

By the late 1990s, brain imaging studies and experiments with rodents had begun to reveal a second previously unknown biological pathway. This pathway was underlying the process of eating for pleasure. Like I wrote before in case of obesity standard regulatory system will tell the brain that we have fat deposits stored for an extended period and that we can endure little hunger. Overeating is a form of drug addiction. What was found was that extremely sweet or fatty food that we have today but were not present in nature, captivate the brain reward circuit in much the same way that cocaine and gambling can do. Even just seeing the food will trigger the brain response. As quickly as such food meets the tongue, taste buds give signals to different areas of the brain. That will result in response that will trigger the release of the neurochemical dopamine. Frequently overeating highly palatable foods saturate the cerebellum with significant amount of dopamine that forces the brain to ultimately adjusts by desensitizing itself, decreasing the number of cellular receptors that identify and respond to the neurochemical. High and constant dopamine level is the form of stimulus that is over excessive, something called supernormal stimuli. It is a term that evolutionary biologists apply to represent the stimulus that will evoke a response more significant than the stimulus for which it evolved, even if it is artificial. The food industry uses it all the time almost in every possible way they can think of. They even try to link emotional responses and feelings of social acceptance and wellbeing with supernormal stimuli.

Consequently, as a resistance build up, people may in truth, proceed to gorge as a process of recollecting or even preserving a sense of well-being. This is possibly the reason why downregulation of leptin receptors in the brain happens also. There was a series of research done from 2007 to 2011, at the University of Gothenburg in Sweden. They proved that the release of ghrelin (the hunger hormone) by the abdomen immediately enhances the discharge of dopamine in the brain's award circuit. This is a significant finding. They also discovered that medications that prevent ghrelin from binding to neurons restrain the tendency for overeating in people who are obese.

Under normal conditions, leptin and insulin suppress the release of dopamine. In theory, this should reduce the sense of pleasure as a meal continues. Recent rodent studies suggest that the brain stops responding to these hormones as the amount of fatty tissue in the body increases. Thus, continued eating keeps the brain awash in dopamine even as the threshold for pleasure keeps going up. A form of maladaptation to our current environment and way of eating and living. If we switch the stimuli from food to cocaine or nicotine or caffeine, we can suppress the hunger drive. Alternatively, also vice versa. If we stop smoking appetite goes up. Tobacco use was linked to hunger suppressing effect even among Pre-Columbian indigenous Americans. Cigarette smoking for weight loss might not be a good idea, because we will swap one addiction to another. You can try extracted nicotine in products like chewing gum or electronic cigarettes with caffeine combination. There is, for example, particular drugs that target the brain hunger center for lowering appetite like Belviq, Contrave, Saxenda, Phentermine, and Qsymia. Phentermine is an amphetamine. Regular "speed" can work also. Anti-seizure drug Topamax for epilepsy and migraine headaches lowers the appetite and is registered to treat the binge eating disorder. If everything else fails, there are seven weight loss surgeries registered so far, from cutting, stapling to ballooning. All because of supernormal stimuli of refined food.

When we see a hamburger, it is supernormal stimuli, or when we see any food item that does not exist in that form in nature especially if it combines any form of fat and carbohydrates or regular sugar together it is supernormal stimuli. Primal urges or instincts effect our behavior and our reptilian brain and basically control us more than we would like to admit. There is a problem of conditioning too. When you spend years working on that promotion or spend years in college and finally get that job or diploma you feel great. It takes time and effort. But when you go to the fridge and open bag of chips you feel great too. Alternatively, you can open that porn site with two clicks of the button and give yourself a most powerful reward that your brain can naturally give itself. However, there is a problem. In nature, we would have to work very hard to get that bite, and it was not salted or filled with fat and sugar. Alternatively, when we wanted to find a mate, we had to be able to fight off other males. We would have to work for it hard for any reward. It would take significant time and effort. However, in the modern era, it is effortless. One phone call to the pizza place one click on a porn button on a mouse, and that is it. Instantaneously we can reward ourselves with pleasure no time or effort needed. Moreover, there are drugs, movies, video games, alcohol, gambling. These things are all form of instant gratification. There are too easy to obtain, and they provide short bursts of pleasure. This conditioning alters our perception and reconfigures our reward centers in the brain. Modern environmental stimulants may activate instinctive responses which evolved before the modern world. When we can get supernormal stimulation all the time effortlessly our brain downregulates the receptors, and we have a problem, we need more. Also, when we do get more, brain will downregulate the receptors some more, and we again need more. It becomes an addictive behavior, before we overdose.

There is a group of sensitive individuals that will respond excessively to delicious foods. They would have to excessive response in the brain reward circuit that will dramatically alter their brain chemistry. Overstimulated brain reward circuit will override any self-control mechanism so that willpower will rarely if ever be sufficient to force them to resist eating those foods once they are around. Researchers at The Scripps Research Institute in Jupiter, Florida found that in rats that have been given unrestricted access to high-calorie foods, their brain showed neurological changes in their reward circuit. High-calorie foods, in this case, were sausage, bacon, cheesecake, and chocolate. It was the first study that showed that the neurological mechanism that drives people into drug addiction is also driving the compulsion for overeating, pushing people into obesity. Some of the rats were given only one hour a day to feast on high-fat foods, while others had unlimited access 24 hours a day. Both groups were given access to a typical, healthy lab rat chow food. The one group that possessed infinite access to high-calorie food ate little to none of the standard bland low-calorie chow alternatives. They quickly had grown obese because they eat as much as they could, about twice the amount of calories as the control. The big surprise was that even the rats that had limited access to junk food did their best to keep up. During that one hour, they ate as much as they can with no stopping. They managed to consume, on average, 66% of their daily calories in the course of that one single hour per day and quickly developed a pattern of compulsive binge eating. It was also observed that a group of obese rats with unlimited access to the junk food had shown severely increased threshold for reward levels. The same thing happens with drug addiction. After showing that obese rats had clear addiction-like food seeking behaviors and that increased threshold for reward levels is forcing them to seek more and more to reach the same level of reward the researchers investigated underlying neurological mechanisms that are responsible for these changes. There is a specific receptor in the brain known to play a significant role in vulnerability to drug addiction, the dopamine D2 receptor. In the brain, there are neurotransmitters like dopamine. Dopamine is a feel-good chemical that will get released when we have some pleasurable experience like sex or food. The D2 receptor responds to dopamine. Cocaine, for example, is the drug that increases dopamine levels in the brain by blocking its retrieval. Overstimulating the dopamine receptors with any supernormal stimuli will eventually lead to neural adaptation in the form of downregulation of the receptors. Also, this was shown in the study too. Levels of the D2 dopamine receptors were significantly reduced in the brains of obese animals. The same thing happens in drug addicts. To determent the level of influence of dopamine in the rats eating behavior, a virus was inserted into the brains of a test group of the animals to knock out their dopamine D2 receptors. Addiction-like behavior happened almost instantly. The next day their brains changed into a state that was consistent with an animal that had been overeating for several weeks. Also, the animals had become compulsive in their eating behaviors. The research that took three years to finish confirms the addictive properties of junk food. A previous 2001 study published in the Lancet also observed a similar death of dopamine receptors in the cerebella of numerous overweight people as in those hooked on cocaine or alcohol. Although their study focused on high-fat foods, full neurochemical and behavioral changes might be due to a combination of both sugar and fat.

Animals binge-eating lipids and animals binge-eating sugars experience different physiological effects, but the most substantial impact can be brought by the combination of neural effects from both of these ingredients. Actually, the most desired food for the lab rats appeared to be a food item with the highest combination of fat and sugar: cheesecake. There is a long line of studies that also have noted links between food and drugs. One team for instance at the University of California, Santa Barbara, found that male rats chose sugar over small amounts of cocaine, while female rats did the opposite. A Swedish team found that ghrelin (hunger hormone) could make rats seek sugar the way addicts seek drugs. A different study from different institute using a mouse model found that 15-week exposure to 60% high-fat diet induces epigenetic silencing of tyrosine-hydroxylase, dopamine reuptake transporter and mu-opioid receptor genes in brain regions associated with reward (nucleus accumbens, ventral tegmental area, prefrontal cortex, and hypothalamus). In one other study at Concordia University in Montreal, they studied rats that had learned to give themselves heroin by pressing a lever. When scientists decided to take away the heroin, the rats after some time mostly stopped pressing the lever. However, when the researchers also took away the rats food, the lever pressing came back with a vengeance. At least in animals, sweet or fatty foods can act a lot like a drug in the brain. The most of the psychologists would also agree that supernormal stimulation influences the behavior of humans as powerfully as that of animals.

In the book, Wasteland: The (R)Evolutionary Science Behind Our Weight and Fitness Crisis, Harvard psychologist Deirdre Barrett had analyzed very well how junk food triggers exaggerated stimulus to natural cravings for salt, sugar, and fats. The issue is that most of the regular people are not psychologists and can't detect this in their own behavior. Supernormal stimuli exist in nature too. When scientists isolate the traits that can trigger certain instincts like colors or shapes or patterns and then applied them to animals, they go behaving extremely instinctively and outside of the normal behavior. Instincts had no bounds. Once the researches isolate the instinctive trigger, they can create greatly exaggerated dummies which animals would choose instead of the realistic alternative. For example, seeing red male stickleback fish would ignore the real rivals and attack wooden replicas with brightly painted underbellies and were even reacting aggressively when red postal van passed the lab window. Songbirds would abandon their eggs that are pale blue dappled with gray and sit on a black polka dotted fluorescent blue dummies so big that they would continuously slide off. They would prefer to feed fake baby birds with more full and redder mouths then their real ones and the hatchlings would ignore their parents to beg for food from fake beaks with more dramatic markings. It is easy to assume that these kind of behaviors reflect some mistake or manipulation but it is far from the truth. The truth is that this is entirely evolutionary justifiable action and will contribute to the survival of the species. The big colorful egg is a symbol of health for a bird so her instinct is correct and it is a conditioned to force her to spare more of her time to go to sit on black polka dotted egg because that egg is having more chances for successful hatching. In nature, there are no mistakes only in the human interpretation of nature.

Birds will never be exposed to technology, so the supernormal stimuli are positive conditioning for the survival of the species. In a technologically driven modern environment, it is a different story. We have not been adequately adapted in the evolutional sense to our modern environment, and the consequences are terrible. For example, obesity is an epidemic and not just obesity, most of our other health problems as well. All of the so-called diseases of affluence are physiological maladaptations in essence. Why? Because pleasure seeking actions in all forms drive most of our behavior. It will make us eat even when we are not hungry in pursuit of pleasure and satisfaction. It will make our brain overstimulated in any possible form and way we can think of. Problem is significant on a population scale and can become even worse in specific individuals that have levels of dopamine receptors that are less expressed. It can make them susceptible to compulsive behavior.

Our physiology is not adapted to be continuously bombarded with supernormal stimuli, to have instant gratification in all forms, never to feel hunger, never to have to do any physical activity, to have a never-ending stream of animal products, sugar, and fat. We act impulsively, emotionally and instinctively like most other animals because we are condition to do it for survival. Like it or not, at the end, this will have lasting health consequences.

Hominin dietary evolution

"The pressure to obtain relatively difficult to find high-quality plant foods encourages the development of mental complexity with is paid for by greater foraging efficacy"-Katharine Milton

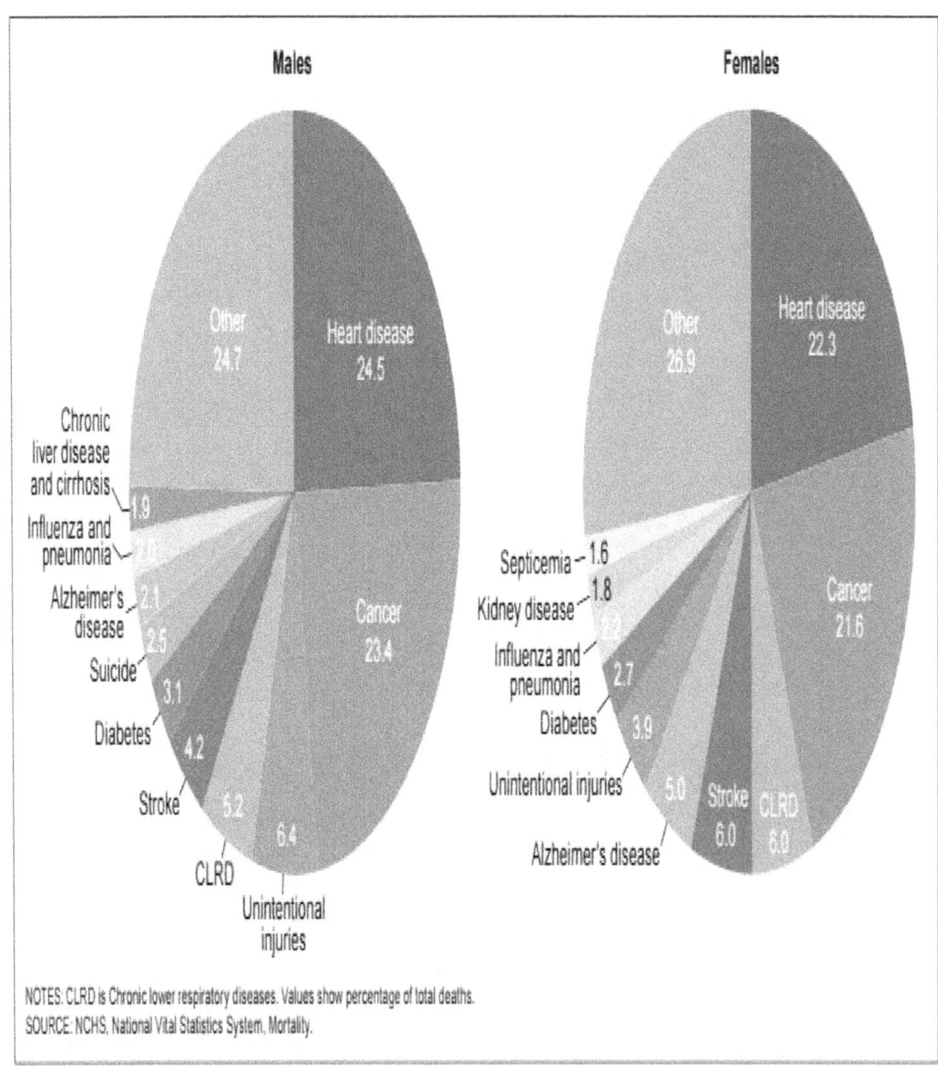

Figure 1. Percent distribution of the 10 leading causes of death, by sex: United States, 2014

Evolution of the hominin diet is an important topic that plays a role in our understanding of our physiology. We have to understand how we came into existence and after that what style of living should we have that is going to be in line with our physiology. If we go too far out in the way we live and eat then we will have to cope with the consequences mostly in the form of health care bills and impaired quality of life. Most of our diseases are caused by diet and lifestyle. People have a hard time believing how many serious health problems are caused by non-evolutionary congruent diet. Every year Center for Disease Control and Prevention updates the list of leading causes of death in the United States and for all other developed countries statistics are very similar. When you are developed as a nation, then you have more money to spend on processed food and meat. In 10 most top leading causes of death, most are caused by life choices. The data is alarming. It is beyond that.

I will try to translate data from the chart to be more clearly understood. When data shows that 24 percent of people are going to die from heart disease what that means is that for example if you have a family of four, one of them will probably die from heart disease and one from cancer. Two left. Then after that, go and take your pick, you have diabetes, stroke, different neurological conditions or liver cirrhosis, crld is 5% (tobacco smoking is by far the most critical risk factor for chronic bronchitis and emphysema, accounting for about 80% of all cases). Normal painless death by natural aging, just forget about it. Doesn't exist anymore. And the problem is not just about the way we are going to die, it is more about when because life expectancy is dramatically shortened and our quality of life is destroyed. We are not going to just drop dead from the cancer. There are going to be a lot of chemotherapy and depression an again cancer goes away then reappears again after a couple of years. When you have a stroke and still manage to survive, you can lose a big chunk of your brain, and before you die from a heart attack, there are going to be a lot of treatments. What treatments include is all the lifestyle changes we do not like plus drugs and surgery. Quitting of smoking, physical activity, maintaining a healthy weight, managing stress (getting upset or angry can trigger a heart attack). After that comes angioplasty (ballooning device is placed through blocked coronary artery with idea to compress the plaque against the wall); bypass of narrowed or blocked coronary arteries; beta-blockers to block the effects of adrenaline and decrease the resting heart rate; calcium channel blockers to relax blood vessels and increase blood flow; diuretics (you may know these as water pills to help flash out water and salt from your tissues and bloodstream). No salting of food makes it easier for our heart to pump. Then something to dilute our blood and something to prevent blood clots like Warfarin. And of course cholesterol-lowering drugs.

Statins are the standard line, and almost all patients will be prescribed one of them but what they do not like to tell is that statistically when we look at real numbers they are only useful in early stages in treating heart disease. They are effective also in those patients that are at elevated risk but still without cardiovascular disease as some sort of prevention. Statins also and that is rarely mentioned have side effects that are no joke. They include muscle pain, the risk of diabetes mellitus and abnormalities in liver enzyme tests. Who wants to be in constant pain? What they in reality do is to block something known as s HMG-CoA. They inhibit the enzyme HMG-CoA that has the crucial role in producing of cholesterol. However, again if you go and eat it blocking enzymes in your own liver and your own production has no point. That means no meat, no eggs, no dairy. If we look at what these diseases do, it is a life of despair.

It is not just:" Well ok I will live the way I like then if I die in 60 instead of 65 who cares, a will die happy." If you think that, you are in dangerous delusion. Today 5-year-old children already have signs of arteriosclerotic plaque with approximately 50% of children having it at 2-15 years-of-age to 85% at 21-39 years-of-age (Atherosclerotic Cardiovascular Disease Beginning in Childhood doi: 10.4070/kcj.2010.40.1.1). Diseases start early and could last for decades before you finally go. The death rate of heart disease and stroke will probably be much higher, but some patients literally get scared to death. And they are right. They are about to die when they hear the news of cardiovascular disease, so some percentage of them do make the lifestyle changes and manage to avoid a heart attack. However, again this is just a chart of diseases that will kill us.

The real, bigger and more advanced chart is the one with the whole list of chronic diseases that would not necessarily kill us, although some can do that too, but will "just" keep our lives in misery. These are so-called chronic diseases like arthritis, asthma, allergies, back pain, Crohn's, osteoporosis, autoimmune conditions like psoriasis, different forms of lupus, multiple sclerosis, wide variety of mental diseases like add, depression, bipolar, epilepsy, addictions of different forms, or just "regular" conditions like anxiety, acne vulgaris, low level of energy and fatigue, sleep, memory and mood issues. Also, something I like to call a trash can diagnosis of Fibromyalgia (if they don't know what is wrong with you then you have Fibromyalgia). In nature there is no free lunch, every action has a reaction direct or indirect one. We cannot escape our choices.

Let me give one example of how chronic diseases occur and progress so that we can start to understand this. The most common nervous system disorder of all neurological disorders is something called essential tremor (ET). It usually involves an involuntary shaking of the arms, hands or fingers but sometimes it can also affect the head, vocal cords or other body parts. It is a different condition then Parkinson's disease but is often misdiagnosed as such. In most severe cases, ET interferes with a person's activities of daily living, like dressing, taking care of personal hygiene, feeding, and is generally progressive in most cases. Some people have it in families so genetics play a role and will develop symptoms at an early age but it is not bad genetics that is the real problem, and I will explain. Prevalence is approximately 4% in people's age 40 and older and significantly higher among individuals in their 60s with an estimated 1 in 5 of individuals in their 90s and over. It is not a normal condition and animals do not have this. What happens is that when you heat amino acids (building blocks of protein) in the presence of creatine and monosaccharide sugars, they have a reaction and amino acids lose their molecular form. What that means is that they are different but not that much, and that is the problem because our body does not recognize them as different. It thinks that they are just regular aminos. Again we are still not fully adapted to our new lifestyle. So what happens is that they start to be incorporated into our cells. Because their molecular structure is different, it causes problems in the form of mutations. Having mutations maybe sounds like a good idea for an SF movie, but in real life it kills. It causes changes to DNA. Meat heated at high temperatures, especially above 300 °F (as in grilling or pan frying), or that is cooked for a long time, tend to form more of these mutated amino acids named heterocyclic amines (HCAs). For example, well done, grilled, or barbecued chicken and steak all have extreme concentrations of HCAs. Chicken is the worst of them all actually, with around two times more of this carcinogen then beef or pork. Marinating meat before cooking in some form of antioxidant-rich marinades like garlic or rosemary seems to help. Garlic at 20 gm/100 gm marinade reduced carcinogen production by about 70%. In contrast, regular barbecue sauce that contains much sugar caused a significant increase in chemical formation, tripling the levels after 15 minutes of cooking. There is a list of different types of these messed up aminos in cooked meat that are created. PhIP (2-Amino-1-methyl-6-phenylimidazopyridine) is the most abundant one. Long-term rodent studies confirmed that PhIP causes mammary gland and colon cancer. The most toxic and mutagenic of all is MeIQ. MeIQ is precisely 24 times more carcinogenic than aflatoxin, and aflatoxin is one of the most toxic substances ever created by mold. All of the other ones, and there are more than 20 HCAs, are more toxic than benzopyrene. Benzopyrene is a primary carcinogen that does the most damage in smokers and is found in cigarette smoke and coal tar.

Smoke actually at the same time during cooking creates a list of other different mutagens named polycyclic aromatic hydrocarbons (PAHs). Cooking techniques that expose meat to smoke or charring contribute to PAH formation. PAHs are created with the high-temperature cooking of meat. For example, when fat and juices from grilled meat drip and cause flames, the fumes will be filled with PAHs that will then adhere to the surface of the meat. Any form of burning can create them, for example, coal, oil, gas, wood, garbage, and tobacco have them too. They are also formed where smoke is used such as smoking of meats. These unnatural mutagens (HCAs and PAHs) that are formed with unnatural activities such as grilling are capable of damaging DNA because of our lack of adaptation to them. There is no known animal in nature except modern humans that grills meat. The body has a line of specific enzymes to neutralize these mutagens. Researchers have discovered that the action of those enzymes differs significantly among people. And that is a problem. In individuals who have lower levels of these enzymes, exposure to these compounds may be associated with an increase in cancer risks. Some of us can cope better with detoxifying these mutagens and some can't and will have a higher risk of cancer.

And that is what is called a genetic factor in medicine. It is not that we are born with bad genes, and that is it, you will get cancer or you will not. The situation is more complicated than that.

Of course, some level of cancer happens in animals too, but 23.4% of all deaths are not from genetics. It is an epidemic of biblical proportions because it is, in essence, a form of maladaptation to our environment. One of the HCAs that is formed is Harmane. Harmane is a neurotoxin that is strongly associated with essential tremor. If exposed by injection mouse will develop an extreme tremor in just 3.1 minutes after the exposure and tremor would last for hours. Because it is fat soluble, it will accumulate over time in all fat tissues including the brain. It is found in elevated levels not just in brains of ET patients but also in Parkinson's disease. When compared to control group Harmane concentration is precisely 50 percent higher in brains of essential tremor patients. It is also elevated in blood samples too. If there is a patient that has a family history of essential tremor blood work result show the highest concentrations of all people. Essential tremor is liver enzyme detoxification disease, a form of maladaptation. People with ET but without family history will have little lower levels then people with family history but still well above normal levels. Elevated Harmane in ET is due to an inherited reduction in the capacity to metabolize it out of the system. Same with any other disease, some people are more prone to it some less, but none of us are immune completely. That is why we see that with time percentage of people with disease goes up. From 4% in the 40s to 20% in 90s. If we managed to live long enough most of us will eventually get it, except for the people who do not consume it. For each additional 10 grams/day of meat consumed, the odds of ET are increased by 6%.

Now you might not get ET, all of this is a just small example for logical understanding. The real difficulty is that there is a long list of different chronic diseases to make a pick from depending on individual genetics. Don't even want to mention the level of cost of medical treatments. When a scientists look at this kind of data for mortality rates and similar things they can correlate factors of behaviors to different diseases. For example, excess cholesterol causes atherosclerosis (fatty deposits that can clog arteries) and then causes heart disease. We do not need dietary cholesterol. Our own liver creates as much as we need so any dietary cholesterol at any time in our entire life, one mg of it is excess that needs to be detoxified. It is done by forcing it to go back to our digestive tract in an assumption that there will be some fiber to bind with it and take it out by excrement. There is no other mechanism that our body can use and if there is no fiber in the digestive system, it will be reabsorbed back to the bloodstream. We cannot detoxify any fat molecule through kidneys only through the colon. Also, no our body does not have to have cholesterol to make every cell in our body, our liver makes all cholesterol we need our entire life every second of it. Why? Because we are not carnivores. Livers of carnivores do not make cholesterol, for them, cholesterol is an essential nutrient. They do not need to because carnivores eat cholesterol in every bite of meat, so they are adapted at eating it by evolution, and we are not. I will hear this all the time how cholesterol is no big deal and usually from the people that are trying to justify their habits. In my view, this is just one example of self-illusion triggered by an underlying subconscious desire for supernormal stimuli. Apparently, everything has to be eaten in "moderation" so a couple of eggs in special occasions or in the period of a month is fine if you have a very clean diet and exercise and clean life in general. The majority of cholesterol leaves the body through the colon. Fecal excretion can occur via two independent pathways by biliary secretion, and by excretion by enterocytes, a mechanism coined as trans-intestinal cholesterol excretion (TICE). Fiber bulks, speeds, and dilutes the intestinal waste stream to facilitate the removal of excess cholesterol from the body.

Eating animal products are associated with shortening life while eating fiber is associated with prolonging life expectancy because our number 1 killer is heart disease and number 3 stroke (basically the same disease as a heart disease just different outcome). If our number one killer is something completely uncorrelated for example bubonic plague like in the Middle Ages and heart disease was on 157th place, then we would not have to be worrying about cholesterol at all, we will have to be worrying about sanitation. At this time in our evolution situation is like it is. Cancer is significantly lifestyle disease too. Genetics play the role, but the lifestyle is as much as important as genetics because of the toxic overload and mutagens form external intoxication and also inherent lack of adequate level of self-repairing autophagy mechanism. The very important risk factor in cancer is chronic inflammation and impaired immune system. Most of the population today have high levels of chronic inflammation. Then there is on wide population scale the lack of some essential micronutrients (essential and some important non-essential micronutrients, not calories) and antioxidants. So in one hand, we have inflammatory compounds, toxins, and mutagens but in another hand lack of micronutrients and antioxidants. Also, then there is a chronic elevation of cancer-promoting hormones like IGF-1 and estrogen.

Just these three diseases are causing more than 50% of deaths, and all three are substantially dependent on a diet. When we look at the list of 15 leading causes of death more than 80% are lifestyle influenced. Everyone in the medical field knows this, all doctors, all scientists, all industries. Well maybe not all of the doctors, some are just bad. Only ones that have a big problem with this is us, regular people because we like the way we live and we would not like to change anything in a way we eat. We will go to MD's if we have any problem right. Well, doctors are just there to do their job of prescribing pills. They are not there to care for you. Only you can take care of you. Problem is you don't want to. You want the pill. We like our dopamine inducing drugs in the form of food and any other variation. The most convenient way would be to find some research that is in a line of what we like and then use it as an excuse. Then we can go to the medical doctor to get some magic pill. There is a good book on the subject called HOW NOT TO DIE by Michael Greger, M.D. It has a lot of practical to do lists but if we do not understand the underlying logic of our behavior patterns then nothing can help us, no practical advice will be enough. Science cannot govern our every act. We must logically govern ourselves and our behaviors in a line of understanding of our history and how we came into existence.

In reality, we need to take a look at the lives of our ancestors and in longer time spread than just the paleo period. Why? Because or physiology is passed, from one species to another. Hominins too had inherited their anatomy from species that came before them. All life on the planet actually can be traced back to single species. How far we need to go? As far as we need to so that we can understand how evolutionary adaptations form. Then we would have a complete picture. Have you ever wonder why scientists do experimentation on mouses? Do you think that physiology of some small creature like a mouse is so different from our own? Oldest fossil ever found on Earth dates back to about 4.2 billion years. It was microscopic bacteria found in the Nuvvuagittuq Supracrustal Belt in Quebec, Canada. These rocks represent some of the first formed sedimentary rocks on Earth, dating back to 4.3 billion years ago. At that time the area was an iron-rich ocean. Bacteria would have lived in hot vents in the 140F (60C) that are similar to iron-oxidizing bacteria found near other hydrothermal vents today. New proposed date for beginning of the life on earth after this discovery is 4.5 billion years. What is interesting is that 4.5 billion years is just one hundred million years after Earth had formed. After first life had formed, it started to evolve. There were also time periods of high and almost total extinction. Three hundred sixty-three million years ago, in Carboniferous Period the Earth had begun to resemble its present state. There was an abundant amount of vegetation with insects and sharks that swim in the oceans as top predators. Four-limbed tetrapod's, the four-limbed vertebrates (from Greek: τετρα- "four" and πούς "foot") slowly developed adaptations which will help them to occupy a terrestrial habitat. Then from amphibians came the first reptiles. Soon following the occurrence of the first reptiles, two branches split off from them. Synapsids (precursors to mammals) had separated from sauropsids (reptiles). It is very likely that synapsids had a direct ancestor to all modern mammals. Today there are still 5,500 species of living synapsids. They include mammals, both aquatic (whales) and flying (bats) species. Humans are also synapsids. During Triassic and Jurassic period these ancestors of living mammals all still had a high metabolic rate. They had to consume food in much higher quantity. To facilitate fast ingestion, these synapsids evolved chewing and specialized differentiated teeth that aided in chewing. These include the molars, canines, and incisors.

After the Permian–Triassic extinction, the synapsids numbers and variety were severely reduced to the point that they did not count more than three surviving clades. One of three surviving clades was the increasingly mammal-like cynodonts. The jaws of cynodonts bear a resemblance to modern mammalian jaws. The cynodonts were carnivorous, herbivorous, and insectivorous and as the Triassic period progressed they became increasingly smaller and more mammal-like. The first mammalian forms evolved from the cynodonts during the early Norian Age of the Late Triassic, about 225 Mya. Early mammals mostly fed on insects. They were small shrew-like animals. Because there is a fossil record as evidence, it is theorized that first mammals already had milk glands for their young and constant body temperature. Mammals had one more unique characteristic that evolved with them, and that is neocortex region of the brain. The starting point of the diet was predominately insects, but they started diversifying almost immediately. In one study at the University of Bristol team of paleontologist led by Pamela Gill found that first mammals had by this time already evolved teeth suited to fit more specialized menus. The animals at the center of the research were Morganucodon and Kuehneotherium. They lived around 200 million years ago, and someone will argue that this period is too long ago and that diet of these animals do not have an impact on our physiology and that is correct. Something we have a hard time understanding is that it took 140 million years for the diet to shift from insects to fruits and leaves. Not 140 thousand years, 140 million years, million.

In an evolutionary sense when we look at for example the paleo diet or something our ancestor eat a couple of thousands of years ago is utterly irrelevant. Physiology does change, but it needs some time to do that. What Gill and colleagues for example found was that the Morganucodon was a hard biter and had a bite about 50% stronger than that of Kuehneotherium. He was able to crash beetles and other hard-shelled prey. Kuehneotherium likely had a softer diet of scorpionflies and early members of the moth lineage. In evolutionary sense, if we have specialized our diet too successfully and we can thrive in the current environment, the problem arises, and we are more likely to perish during a mass extinction because we are eating only one thing. If we have different species that are accustomed to different niches and can eat just about anything and 90 percent of food goes away, there will still be some left that will live on scraps. By the 85 million years ago, they have already diversified their diet. These variations in the diet may hold a key for providing circumstances that allowed them to survive in the mass extinction that happened around 66 million years ago. It was at the end of the Cretaceous Period. About 85 million years ago, is when a group of arboreal, small and nocturnal insect-eating mammals called the Euarchonta (meaning true ancestors) had begun the speciation that will lead to the primate, tree shrew and flying lemur orders. The term Euarchonta is a proposed grand order of mammals, and their diet was still based on insects. In the next 20 million years, the modern forms of mammalian orders arose after the great extinction of non-avian dinosaurs.

Stem-primates first appear in the fossil record between 65 and 55 million years ago. They may have been the first mammals to have fingernails in place of claws. One of the early stem-primates is Plesiadapis that existed about 58–55 million years ago. Plesiadapis possessed claws and had the eyes still located on each side of the head. This made them faster on the ground but allowed them to go to the top of the trees still. In time, they began to spend longer periods on lower branches of trees, feeding on fruits and nuts. So at the 60 Mya mark, our ancestor species had started to eat plants. In time interval to 60 Mya evolution have diversified from eating just insects and living on the ground to fruits, nuts, and insects omnivorous diet and semi-living on trees. One other of semi-primates named Carpolestes simpsoni was more like the living primates with grasping digits allowing him to have a firm grip on branches but no forward-facing eyes. Dental morphology of C. simpsoni showed more specially adapted diet specialized for eating fruit, seeds, and invertebrates.

Next 10 to 20 Ma is approximately the time period when diet completely shifted. Eocene Epoch (55.8-33.9 million years ago) matches with the appearance of the first species of the placental mammals. These orders or in other words their descendants are still present today. Primates diverged into two suborders Strepsirrhini (wet-nosed primates) and Haplorrhini (dry-nosed primates). The Haplorrhini liver was the first one that lost the ability to make its own vitamin C. What this in reality means is that they have been eating too much of the plant foods already that their bodies decided to turn off production of the vitamin C to save the energy. All of their descendant species had to include fruit in the diet because vitamin C must be obtained externally. Also, this is a significant factor. Humans today too must obtain vitamin C or we will suffer and die from scurvy. What this means is that already the early primates were dependent on plant foods on such level that their liver discontinued producing vitamin C. In carnivores species, because they eat only meat vitamin C is produced internally, and it is not a vitamin for them. When we start to consume plants and we start to consume them in a constant manner evolution shuts down everything that is not necessary. So this can tell us a lot about a diet of early primates. They transmuted to fruits and leaves instead of insects and became almost wholly herbivores. This is the adaptation that took tens of millions of years to complete. I would estimate it to be more than 30 million years that had passed from insect-eating Euarchonta to the Haplorrhini.

What happened then is a process of natural selection that strongly favors traits that enhance the efficiency of foraging. Hence, as plant foods became increasingly important over time adaptation gradually gave rise to the group of characteristics presently considered as the property of primates. Most of these traits are adapted to facilitate the movement and foraging in trees. For example, adaptation yielded hands well suited for grasping branches and manipulating slender and small fruit and leaves. In order to detect ripe fruits and enable safe moving through arboreal habitat adaptation forced improvement of the optical capabilities (including depth perception, sharpened acuity, and color vision). Good vision is crucial for moving through the three-dimensional space of the forest canopy and to quickly determine the appearance of ripe fruits or tiny, young leaves.

Moreover, such environmental pressures also favored the ability to learn and remember the identity and locations of edible plant parts and also to calculate the optimal foraging strategies to save energy thus increasing behavioral flexibility as well. Foraging benefits from the improvement of visual and cognitive skills. As a result, it promoted development of an unusually large brain, a characteristic of primates since their inception. Eating meat or bone marrow had nothing to do with the development of the larger brain.

Katharine Milton was studying the foraging behavior of howler and spider monkeys in the Republic of Panama. Her studies led to looking at the diet of primates and their evolution leading to the evolution and diet of humans as well (Diet and Primate Evolution-Scientific American 16, 22 - 29, 2006). When we think of hunting, we usually think of animal pray. Plants cannot run, so how would they defend? Usually, the most damage to the plant is done by insects and herbivores, so plants have developed a different array of poisons. Plants are also attacked just like us by fungus and bacteria and another kinds of microorganisms. These poisons also have their porpoise as insecticides and fungicides and even herbicides like caffeine. Caffeine is a natural herbicide in leaves of the coffee plant. Leaves eventually fall on the ground, and that will at the end even kill the coffee plant root itself. In a way, coffee plant commits suicide after a period of time when the concentration of caffeine in the ground reach the toxic level. All of these chemicals are a natural part of the plants. These chemicals can also taste awful, at worst, they can be lethal. On another hand, some of them are very beneficial for us because they act as anti-fungal and anti-microbial substances when we eat them like oil of oregano for example and can have the positive impact on our immune system and have numerous other positive effects. The common name for them is phytochemicals from Greek word phyton, meaning plant. Also, plant cells are enclosed by walls made up of materials collectively referred to as fiber. Fiber is sturdy and can resist breakdown by mammalian digestive enzymes and don't provide energy in the form of sugar. Many people think that for us fiber is a waste of time and digestion because it does not provide any energy. However, that is not true. Fiber has a different positive impact on our system in the form of detoxifying and feeding probiotic bacteria, but it is not a viable energy source.

Different plant foods will lack different nutrients we need. For example, one plant may have some but not all amino acids and vitamins in an adequate level, or even if it is nutrient dense and don't have fiber it may lack energy in the form of carbohydrates (starch and sugar). Mammals that depend primarily on plants for meeting their daily nutritional requirements and are not adapted for one particular plant food source that is in abundance as a consequence must seek out a variety of complementary food sources from a different array of plants. They have to combine different food types to get all of the nutrients they need. This demand greatly complicates food gathering. It is a tough life, and it is a constant struggle for food and requires constant use of thinking. Most arboreal hominids and other primates concentrate on ripe fruits on one side and young leaves. They eat other types of food too, but these two are the main ones. Fruits tend to be rich in energy in the form of fructose and relatively low in fiber, but they might not provide all of the essential amino acids and tend to be the rarest of all plant sources. This kind of scarcity complicates things because if in a certain period of the year there are no fruits available. In that time period, the energy requirement is not met, and there is a need for supplementation with different plant sources. Leaves are full of protein and are everywhere, but they are of lower quality meaning there are no carbohydrates in them and we cannot live on them alone, and they tend to be filled with undesirable toxic chemicals. Because primates are not adapted for digesting fiber they eat young leaves that are softener then the tough old ones that cannot be digested. When trees exhibit seasonal peaks in the production of the fruits and young leaves primates have to eat them as much as they can and reliance on a single food choice is not sustainable.

From an evolutionary view, there are two basic strategies for coping with these problems. One is to increase the efficiency of nutrient extraction from fibrous foods. This is a form of adaptation that we can see in mammals that are grazers. For all primate species, eating copious amounts of fiber does not enlist many benefits. For hominids in the past and also for primates, and humans fiber essentially go through their stomach unchanged. Another biological adaptation that can facilitate survival on low-quality plant food is to grow larger over time. When an animal goes larger compared to the smaller animals, it will consume greater overall amounts of food to feed their more extensive tissue mass. However, for reasons that the science had not been able to entirely explain, the more massive the animal is the less calories it needs to sustain itself and attain adequate nourishment. In mathematical terms, larger animals need less energy per unit of body weight. What this means is that larger animals are able to eat less and can eat lower quality food to meet their energy requirements. However, growing bigger for primates is not an option because they are arboreal animals. For growing too massive, they risk falling to their death. So another evolutional strategy is open to arboreal plant eaters and is more behavioral than biological.

It is a foraging strategy. Because fruits are rare and very sporadically scattered in tropical forests, strategy requires the implementation of practices that promise to reduce the energy of acquiring these resources. In order to survive the primates must use their brains more and more to form foraging strategies that are sustainable. A good memory would significantly improve the approach. Ability to recall the exact places of plants that produce desirable fruits and when these trees were likely to bear ripe fruits and to remember the precise directions to these trees would improve foraging profitability in energy expenditure sense by lowering search and travel energy costs by enlarging brain capacity to remember and to plan in advance.

In comparison, grazers do not need brain development because their food is all around them and all they need is to lower their head. Reliance on a memory and foraging strategies have pushed for selection and development of bigger brains that have higher ability for storing information. As a group, primates have always depended on selective feeding and on having the brain power to carry off this strategy successfully. The growth of the brain in combination with growth in body size and a decline in the teeth size supports the notion of a high-quality diet. And this is an evolutionary adaptation that is universal to all primates in the last 66 Ma. Some have gone far like humans. We have brain evolved enough to create pure refined white sugar. Most other plant-eating species, in opposition, have tended to focus heavily on physiological adaptations for better digesting the fiber in order to reduce the need to invest energy for searching for high-quality food. Behavioral adaptations, requiring increased brain power, enable certain species to choose high-quality food. If we look calorie wise, the brain is the most expensive organ to maintain. It takes over the vast amount of energy from food, roughly 20% at rest in humans. Natural selection is not going to favor the development of a massive brain if it is not going to get any benefits from enlargement. The appearance of modern humans with big and capable brains occurred because natural selection favored adaptations that focused on the efficiency of foraging. That was the line of evolution that permitted primates to focus their feeding on the most energy-dense, low-fiber diets they could find and find is a crucial word.

Finding high-quality food in a scarce environment is what created modern humans. It had little to do with eating meat or any other form of energy. A form of energy is of the lesser importance than the way that energy is obtained. In other words, if the meat had anything to do with the development of the brain power, then all of the carnivore species on this planet will be colonizing outer reaches of the galaxy by now. There is no magic nutrient in the meat that was responsible for the rise of the human brain power. Meat is just meat, another energy source. There is no absolute correlation between meat-eating and intelligence. The manner of combining some amount of foraged meat to the predominantly vegan diet did not become a pivotal force in the emergence of modern humans. Also, it is not even correlated to the brain size either. There is no particular relationship among brain size and intelligence; it is more complicated than that. Human adults have around 3 pounds of brain weight, dolphins have 3.5 pounds, an elephant is around 10.5 and sperm whale around 17.2 pounds. Predators as a general rule tend to have a relatively larger brain then the animals they prey upon. Placental mammals also tend to have larger brains than marsupials such as the opossum. There is formula known as encephalization quotient (EQ) for measuring the species brain size related to expectations based on its expected body size. Through the entire evolution of Homo sapiens, the prevailing trait was a steady increase in brain size. It is the truth that much of that size can be attributed to the corresponding increases in body size. Neanderthals, for instance, and many people do not know this used to have larger brains than modern Homo sapiens. What is more important than just the size is how the brain is wired and neuron count.

What is unique for the human brain is that neuron count in one specific part of the brain called cerebral cortex is much higher than in any other animal on the Earth. The human brain has 86 billion neurons if we count them all; 69 billion in the cerebellum; 16 billion in the cerebral cortex and 1 billion in the brain stem and its extensions into the core of the brain. Cerebellum orchestrates essential bodily functions and movement and is a primitive part of the brain, or let's say essential part. The cerebral cortex is the brain's thick corona, the real deal. It is responsible for self-awareness, language, problem-solving, sophisticated mental talents and abstract thought. If we want to measure the intelligence of the species, then we need to count neurons in cerebral cortex. That is it. It is that simple. For example, the elephant brain is three times the size of our own, has 251 billion neurons in its cerebellum, which is needed to manage its massive trunk, but only 5.6 billion in its cortex. Also to be clear an elephant is considered to be highly intelligent species. If we look at the great apes, we are the winner. We have 16 billion neurons in our cortex, but I only was referring to great apes. Homo sapiens appear to have the most significant number of cortical neurons from all species on Earth. Oh, wait. I just lied. We are not the smartest one. The long-finned pilot whale is. His neocortical brain part contains substantially more neurons and glial cells than the neocortex of other large-brained species including humans (Quantitative relationships in delphinid neocortex doi: 10.3389/fnana.2014.00132). So what are we going to do now? We are the species that are more intelligent than any other if we only count land-based animal species, and we have arms and legs and speech so that we can build technology, but guess what, by these measurements, we are not the most intelligent species on Earth. The long-finned pilot whale is. The highest number of neuron in the cerebral cortex is what makes species intelligent. Primates evolved a way to pack far more neurons into that area then other mammals did. The great apes are tiny compared to elephants and whales, yet their cortices are far denser. Orangutans and gorillas have 9 billion cortical neurons, and chimps have 6 billion. So by these measures, humans are 44% more intelligent than orangutans for example because we have 16 billion neurons and they have 9. So if average IQ in humans is 100, the IQ of orangutans would be 56. Chimpanzees fall within the 35-50 range usually. Not bad at all.

Even the small monkeys are very intelligent and more intelligent than their counterpart in size. When we need to think every time we need to eat, it forces the brain to develop for foraging strategies. Let me give an example. In places like South Africa or India, there are a large number of urban monkeys. These wild animals came by their own will to the cities in search for food. In their view, we are just another monkey species. They are not afraid of us at all. They consider us to be non-frightening because we are slower than them and in no small extent weaker, and we have all those food laying around everywhere. So for wild monkeys, it is easier to forage for food in the human environment. Stray dogs do it by sniffing food out, they use their noses, but monkeys use their brains to do the same. Because of the movies and culture average North American is likely to think that monkeys are sweet and cute animals with whom they can have fun with and are super cute when wearing human clothes. In real life, they are everything except cute. For example, they are known to roam neighborhoods in gangs. Baboon gangs run wild in parts of the world like Suburban South Africa. They travel in a flock of around 30, and all of them move following the leader but are so vast apart that it is difficult to stop them sliding into built-up areas.

They can cross walls and roofs at speed. Gangs always have the leader, and they go into foraging for your stuff. Breaking and entering, aggressive behavior and stealing. Regular thug life and it is not funny at all. They break into people houses to steal food, break into cars, they know how to open the doors or anything else for that manner. If they see you do it, they can do it too. They are very intelligent.

Let's think about this. Small brain monkeys can see you use technology and then they can start to use it also for themselves. They learn by themselves how to open windows, how to open doors of cars and fridges and apartments, they can sneak behind your back and steal, and they can unzip zippers and so on. They are not just self-conscious they are conscious of your way of thinking so they can put themselves in your position and predict how you are going to react so that they can manipulate you. I am not kidding. They are known to sneak behind your back and steal stuff, and they are known to lure you out. One of them will steal in front of you and will start to run and when you go outside to chase him off other monkeys that you did not see will go in and steal stuff while you are chasing that one off. And if that is not enough, they are just going to take it out of your hands physically. If you have the problem with that, then they are going to slap you right in the face. They are not afraid of us. And we can say that that is bad enough, but there is more. When they are bored, they are just going to hang out around people and pleasure themselves. The deputy mayor of New Delhi died from a monkey attack. Not directly, they did not attack him, but he tripped off his balcony while trying to fight them off from his apartment. They are aggressive, and they are intelligent. According to one study (Orthographic processing in baboons, Science, 336:245-8, 2012.), baboons have no known language or anything similar but were able to separate real English words from nonsense sequences of letters accurately. If baboons have a physical capability to speak, they will have a real written language because they have the adequate intelligence for it because the ability to distinguish real words from non-real one is the first step in the reading process.

Monkeys like to drink alcohol too. They commonly steal liquor from stores or houses. They even drink in the wild if they can find it and they love it. In one example scientists looked at a group of booze-loving apes in order to find a correlation with human behavior and why humans enjoy drinking it. They studied wild chimpanzees for over 17 years in town named Bossou, Guinea, West Africa. What they observed is repeated drinking of fermented palm sap using a leafy tool as a sponge. The study, called (Tools to tipple: ethanol ingestion by wild chimpanzees using leaf-sponges), watched 51 fermented drinking incidents including 13 chimpanzees between 1995 and 2012. Both humans and African apes share a genetic mutation that allows them to metabolize ethanol efficiently. There is theory called "drunken monkey hypothesis" that states that natural selection favored those hominids that had an affinity to rotten fruit as well. Ethanol or alcohol or rotting fruit was associated with proximate benefits meaning increasing caloric gains. We can extract energy from alcohol. Most of the other species on Earth cannot. It is the unavoidable consequence of a frugivorous diet because after fruits fall to the ground, they start to ferment very quickly. Humans and other primate's attraction to alcohol are derived from the behavior of our ancestors that were eating fermented fruit. Our common ancestor was not averse to ingesting putrefying fruits containing ethanol. Some of the chimpanzees at Bossou consumed significant quantities of alcohol. They displayed behavioral signs of severe inebriation, and some drinkers had to rest after binge drinking fermented sap. Drinking sessions occurred at various times of the day, and there was no disparity among both females and males. Researchers that examined these events sad that, unlike other examples of primates ingesting alcohol, such as green monkeys targeting tourist cocktails in the Caribbean (example: Weird Nature - BBC animals-documentary) the chimpanzee's attraction to fermented palm sap at Bossou was not a result of provisioning by local people. Chimpanzee attraction to fermented palms does not result from hunger either. It is a result of their desire for alcohol as a substance and not as a food source. In nature, Lemurs are known to get high and not in the form of the accident but in the form of intelligent action designed to get themselves into a blissful state. They seek out a particular species of large red millipedes that excrete a form of neurotoxin. Lemurs will bite the millipede gently, and the toxins will cause the lemurs to salivate and then they will rub both the saliva and millipede into their furs as a form of insecticide. They can rub the millipede without biting it, but no, they are suspiciously enthusiastic about the whole process. Chemicals appear to send them into a trance-like state, and they cannot seem to get enough. After they are completely wasted then millipede is a thrown back on the ground or past to another lemur. Dolphins are well known for getting high too. They play around with a puffer fish which, if provoked, releases a nerve toxin. After subsequent biting the puffer gently without harming it and passing it around, they will begin to act "strange."

In another story that BBC reported in Kenya the monkeys where unrestrained, drunken frat boy villains. In the little Kenyan settlement of Nachu, something like a big village, about 300 monkeys were making a practice of robbing the village's produce on a daily basis. The monkeys were typically afraid of males, but have taken to mocking the women and sexually harassing them while they tried to save the grain out in the fields. "The monkeys grab their breasts, and gesture at us while pointing at their private parts. We are afraid that they will sexually harass us", was a quote from villager Mrs. Njeri. The villagers first tried to scare them by making the scarecrows, but that did not work. They are not birds, and they do not feel frightened by humans. So they did not fall on that and where intelligent enough to see through the manipulation. All joking aside villagers had reported that the monkeys had killed livestock and guard dogs, which had left them living in fear, especially for the safety of their babies and children. Monkeys are not easily controlled like other animals, and in this case, all attempts have failed. They have lookouts on the vantage points to warn the others of impending attacks and are smart enough to evade the traps. Poisoning of food did not do anything because they snub the poisoned food away. Kenya

Wildlife Service warned the residents not to kill any of the monkeys, as it is a criminal offense. The government did ultimately send in a unit to observe the monkeys, and since it is illegal to shoot them, they relocated them somehow. Compared to average grazer even with the larger brain size the intelligence difference is significant, and it is not because of the diet difference, it is because the way of acquiring that diet is much more difficult for monkeys. For them and for all primates and our hominin ancestors, it is the hard life that forced development of the brain, not the magic ingredient in food or meat.

Let's compare for example species of herbivorous monkeys with carnivorous species of the approximately same size. In the documentary "Animals Like Us" filmmakers documented kidnaping of wild dog puppies by baboons and raising them in their own baboon tribe as members or pets. Baboons and dogs have similar sizes. The clip of the series which was filmed in a garbage dump near Ta'if, Saudi Arabia, shows a male baboon dragging a puppy away from its den as it screams for its mother. Stolen dogs grow up with the baboon species, like a family member or a member of a group. They were eating with them, sleeping and moving together. The baboons will groom and play with them, and that is important. Baboons only play with family members. The relationship seems to benefit both dog and baboon. The domesticated feral dogs do the same job that they have in human society, and that is to guard the territory. They keep wild dog packs away from monkeys at night while they sleep and in return, they are treated with love and care just like humans would a family pet. Note that in this situation it is important to understand that dogs had more of the equal status in the tribe, they were not pets as monkeys did not feed them. Dogs are carnivores and would eat dump rats and other small animals and meat that they can find. They would not eat fruits and vegetables and other grains and other food on dump yard of plant origins that baboons would eat. There was no direct competition for food thus they have the common tribe in a symbiotic relationship. Now, this video made a lot of controversies. People have a hard time accepting human-like behavior in animals because of our self-image. Was there actual familiar bond happening between the baboons and dogs, again, we will not know until there's real and scientific research done. There is one more video featuring a baboon manhandling a puppy that popped up. A Cornell student named Luke Seitz filmed it. He was on the bird research trip in Ethiopia when he recorded the similar situation of baboon carrying a dog around "like a pet." He also seemingly observed this behavior over a period of days, so it was not just a fluke.

In another case in Guassa plateau, Ethiopia primatologist Vivek Venkataraman observed a remarkable scene: wolves and monkeys casually commingling. In normal circumstances, monkeys are prey, but in this situation, wolves did not seem to have an interest in eating baboons. Baboons and especially young ones are easy prey for the wolves. In fact, they appeared to do everything they could to evade any confrontation. They were ignoring each other and spending hours wandering around through the large gelada herds foraging for rodents. Because they do not compete for a primary food source and attacking the large monkey colony would result in war and bad thing happening to both of them they cohabitate. Humans and wild cats had this kind of arrangement. Domestication of wild cats happened at the same time in the Middle East and Egypt. Wild cats started to spend a lot of time in human villages. There were many rats present because of the grain stores accumulation after the domestication of wild plants. It was the same symbiotic relationship. We used wild cats to lower the rats count; it was beneficial to us to tolerate them. We didn't feed them directly. Also, rats can attract other predators like snakes, and that can be deadly. Thus we tolerated wild cats, and wild cats tolerated us because we are the source of their new food abundance and in time domestication happened. Monkeys are known for adopting people too.

As a young child of just five years old, Marina Chapman was abducted. A possible reason was to ask for ransom, but when criminals did not get any, they just abandoned her in the Columbian jungle. For some five years as a child, she lived out in the wild. She says that she was taken in by a group of capuchin monkeys. These type of monkeys are known to accept young children into their fold. She learned how to forage for food by copying them. She says monkeys taught her how to do it but in any case, she survived. She returned to the human civilization when she was picked up by hunters and sold to a brothel (at that point she was not able to speak the human language). She eventually managed to escape from the brothel, lived on the streets and in the end became a slave of the mafia family.

We are not the only intelligent species and when we look at baboons and dogs one herbivore, another carnivore the baboons are smarter by far. Moreover, the dog itself is a very smart animal. It is a great dogma in science that somehow the newly incorporated meat source equal to a couple of percent of total calories consumed in the form of bone marrow in early hominin diet developed our big brain and that meat is essential to our intelligence and has to be an integral part of the modern diet. Let us look at how developed we actually are before we analyze what made us human and what is our correct diet.

In the 1970s in between 1974 and 1978, there was a tribal war that was raged in Tanzania that started after the death of the local tribe leader. There was the split in the tribal community, and two rival factions were formed. The two tribes involved in the bloodshed were the Kasekela the northern tribe, and the Kahama, the southern tribe that was smaller in number than the northern one. The two tribes emerged from one more prominent tribe as a result of leadership conflict after the death of a senior leader. The first strike began on January 7, 1974. Why the group separated is not clear. A senior leader male Leakey died at the end of 1970. After his death, another male named Humphrey became the leader. He was weak and had two ambitious brothers Carlie and Hugh. Hugh was his competition, and split became so big that rest of the tribe start to take a side. One went with following Humphrey, forming the larger Kasekela tribe, but other tribe members went with Charlie and Hugh forming the smaller Kahama tribe. It was possible to predict which tribe individuals will join by looking at their preferred social contacts before the split. Everything got a sinister turn in 1974 when six Kasekela males attacked and killed a young Kahama named Godi. The battle began. Over four years Humphrey's tribe destroyed his brother tribe, and the seven rebel males died or vanished. The Kasekela began to invade the territory of the smaller tribe systematically. Groups of males would slip into rebel territory and savagely kill a single male in the ambush. They annihilated an entire community that way. Cupping the victim's head as they lay bleeding with blood pouring and then drinking the blood, twisting a limb, standing upright to hurl a four-pound rock, hitting, again and again the stricken and quivering individual, tearing pieces of skin and flesh, just horrific pictures. These gruesome events were even more disturbing because the two tribes had been united just a few years before. The victims were individuals they had known or even been in family ties with and had been traveling with, playing with and growing up with. Of the females from Kahama, two went missing, one was killed, and three were beaten and kidnapped by the Kasakela males and systematically raped as slaves. The Kasakela then prospered to take over entire Kahama's former territory. These territorial gains were not permanent. With the Kahama gone, the smaller remaining Kasakela's tribe had a lot more territory but not enough power to hold it. Their new territory now was directly bordering more prominent tribe, called the Kalande. After some violent skirmishes along their border with superior strength and numbers of the Kalande small Kasakela was forced to retreat and gave up much of their newly gained territory. In history, this incident had been known as the Four-Year War of Gombe. The unusual pattern regarding this war was that it was like stories from early human history or backstabbing in Senate of Ancient Rome or history of Europe's old aristocratic elite. The thing is that this war was waged by our closest living relatives, the chimps.

Before the 1960s, there had been little effort into studying the behavior of the great apes in the wild. To learn more about social structures of early human ancestors that were presumably similar in behavior to the great apes of today a prominent paleontologist in Africa, Dr. Louis Leakey decided to create a study of primate societies. He hired three students to the task: one was assigned to Borneo to investigate orangutans, another one was assigned to Rwanda to investigate gorillas. Jane Goodall, the third one, was assigned to Gombe Forest in Tanzania to investigate chimpanzees. In the extended period of the next five decades, Jane Goodall uncovered much about the behavior of chimpanzees. Many of the findings had not been known before. One of the examples is that they form social structures that were uncannily like our own. They bound with each other in order to form tightly-knit social groups based on social standing and self-interest and also create complex political structures that were based on alliances and partnerships. They had a comprehensive knowledge and understanding of their natural surroundings and were able to utilize them intelligently, even the plants that had medicinal properties when they needed them. One of the areas that were formerly thought to be exclusively human because it requires a high level of brain development is an ability to make and use tools. The chimps were able to make, stripped twigs for termite fishing, stone hammers for nut cracking and sharpened wooden spears for hunting bushbabies. Also, that was not all. Knowledge of making tools was passed from generation to generation creating local cultures, with each troop. It was believed that chimpanzees are strictly vegetarian. Discovery that they are capable of organizing themselves into hunting parties that would carefully stalk and kill colobus monkeys as food made them more human than many in the scientific community would like. Therefore, Goodall faced some criticism. There were claims that she is not objective and is too emotionally involved allowing anthropomorphism to influence her scientific judgment.

They were right to some extent. Before they came to Africa and did real observations she and almost all of her colleagues had this kind of idea that chimps are hairy peaceful little people. Something similar to peaceful hippie communes that have a calm life in harmony with Mother Nature and that they are not like evil, destructive warmongering humans. The disillusionment came in 1974 when war came. To see how much actual intelligence chimpanzee poses let us look at their war tactic. The Kasakelas appeared to be applying a calculated tactic which used the advantage of chimpanzee ecology. In normal conditions, chimps are very social animals. The only thing that they do not do together is to forage for food. When it is time to forage, every chimp is on its own. When it comes to finding food, each adult men and female is on his or her own. Chimps forage for edible plant foods in the surrounding forest, and the usual pattern is that every morning each individual will disperse from others returning to the group later in the afternoon. The Kasakela males created a war strategy. They seemed to be intentionally entering Kahama territory in force just in time to catch lone individuals foraging for food. That penetration of territory by force helped them to isolate the victim so that they can kill the sole individual without the possibility of a larger defense force forming and engaging them. That strategy minimized possibility for adequate response and basically won the war. Separated from their troop during feeding time there is a small chance of surviving. This strategy made a separated individual vulnerable to attack. It was classic guerrilla warfare. For Goodall, the disillusionment was devastating. One particular incident affected her more than others. There was a young male named Satan, ironically. When dying Kahama male with injuries to the face was bleeding to death, Satan was cupping his palms to seize the blood flowing from his face, so that he could drink it. When Goodall published on her observations and research of the Gombe War, her report was not accepted in the scientific community and was not even universally believed. The scientific knowledge at that time did not accept that naturally occurring war between chimpanzees can happen because the war requires human-level intelligence. She was accused of excessive anthropomorphism. Others suggested that her presence had created violent conflict in a naturally peaceful society. However, in later years more extensive research using less intrusive methods had been done.

Today it is accepted, and it is confirmed that chimpanzee societies in their natural state do wage war. Chimpanzee wars are rare, and in general, violence is rare, but it can happen in certain conditions. When it does happen, it can be extreme in its brutality. Male chimps that fall foul of the community hierarchy, for example, have been found disemboweled and castrated for their insubordination. However, it goes both ways. In one observed incident in Tanzania in 2011, four low-ranking beta males joined forces and killed the alpha male. Females do not escape the violence either. It was observed in some areas of Uganda that they are routinely beaten by the males they mate with. These beatings are a form of preventative aggression in order to stop the females from choosing another mate. Females themselves can also be aggressive. During Gombe War, Jane Goodall's team saw a mother-and-daughter duo steal and then kill and eat baby chimp. What was even worse they did it from their own tribe from member they have social interactions with. This was not an isolated incident. In other areas of Uganda, females have also been seen killing an infant. Chimps have been acknowledged to engage and kill humans, too. In Virunga National Park in the Democratic Republic of the Congo, chimps reportedly killed ten people in 2012. Ongoing pressures between the chimps and humans that interact with their habitat may have triggered the killings. Chimps are territorial, and they do not like some humans messing with their territory. All of this also suggests that chimps and humans are cut from the same cloth, unlike some other apes.

For example, there are one other species called bonobo. The bonobo is a different species although related to chimpanzee. They split away from the common chimp about a million years ago (long after human ancestors did). Unlike chimpanzees, they are very peaceable and are closely related to us as chimps. Their peaceful coexistence may be a consequence of ecologically richer habitat with better access to easily digestible food. In such conditions, there is a reduced chance of conflicts over resources. Dominant females, not males run bonobo tribes, and they take "make love, not war" to a whole another level. Sex is practiced not just as a group bounding practice to bond the members of the group together but also as a way to lower the aggression. They will have sex with neighboring troops also to ease tensions or to avoid conflicts. Because the bonobo environment is ecologically more productive than that of the chimpanzees, in essence, there is no necessity to fight over food. When we think of chimps, we have to take another approach than the stupid monkeys one. When we look at our hominin ancestors, we have to take another approach then wild primates or stupid Neanderthals one.

To prove the point, I will mention one more experiment. There was an old saying that money is the root of all evil, a system that tricks people into putting energy outside of themselves, to chase after money instead of searching for the vast riches that lie within. Wright? Is this human nature, or does money corrupt? In a Yale-New Haven Hospital laboratory, capuchin monkeys were taught to use the money. Researchers did not have any particular goal in mind. They just decided to give a monkey a dollar and see what would happen. Instead of the paper money, however, a silver disc with a hole in its center was used, similarly to old Chinese silver coins. After a couple of months of training capuchins realized that they could trade such a token for food. After they realized that, each animal was administered 12 tokens to decide on how to spend it. Food was valued at different prices with different quality like grapes and jelly. The Adam Smith, predicted in one of his theories, that monetary exchange would be restricted only to human beings. We can say now that he was wrong. The capuchin has a small brain. It is a small animal about the size of a human baby. They are not as smart as chimpanzees and other larger primates. Researchers observed that capuchin monkeys actually understood the underlying logic of money and were not just trained to use it. The monkeys understood very well how to budget with money without any training. Researchers changed the market and put jelly at a lower price. Monkeys started to buy more jelly and less grape. Consequently, now we can positively scientifically prove the fact that monkeys are able to ration with prices and money. They behaved precisely like the modern fundamentals of economics say humans will act. The only difference was that they were impulsive and not even a single monkey was able to save any of the tokens. Some scientist theorized that because monkeys steal on regular bases they did not save any from fear of being robbed or were afraid to lose them. The data generated by the capuchin monkeys make them statistically indistinguishable from most stock-market investors. However, yes there was stealing too. Most of them tried to steal some more when the researchers handed them. To contradict this, the tokens were given to the monkeys by inserting one by one through the particular chamber. On one occasion capuchin monkey managed to grab the whole plate of the tokens and chaos broke loose. Capuchin grabbed the plate then make a run for it with a tray filled with tokens and eventually ended up back with all of the other monkeys tossing all the coins to the neighboring cell. Other monkeys grabbed as many coins as they could in effect creating a bank heist. Which is exciting, but not as impressive as what happened next. Not all of the monkeys were lucky enough to get coins. The ones that didn't get any started to look for ways of getting them. What's perhaps the most obvious pattern of one's hold upon currency is the idea that money has intrinsic value. You can use currency to exchange for goods or services or anything else, not just for food. Well, one of the researchers, through the whole turmoil situation, witnessed how one of the monkeys traded money with another one for sex. Following the finishing of the act, the monkey which was paid quickly used it to buy a grape.

The point is that evolution did not begin with the emergence of modern humans in a way it stopped there because modern humans exist only three hundred thousand years. That is an insignificant number in evolutionary terms. After the great extinction of non-avian dinosaurs, first modern forms of mammals had appeared 66 million years ago. They climbed to the trees and became herbivorous. To the time of significant climate change toward the end of the Pliocene, they lived on threes evolving on fruit and green leaves and flowers. They have grown in size and intelligence. That was the period of 60 Ma. Most of our brain, body, and genetics, evolutionary biology and physiology evolved on a trees. One important genus in our family, Australopithecus, emerged in Africa more than 4.5 million years ago, during the Pliocene. In the Pleistocene, the last species of them went extinct. They were bipedal, their brains were not appreciably more massive than those of today's apes, but the brain of today apes are as we have seen pretty human-like. So the evolution in scale was significant from early mammals, and it lasted 60 Ma. The fossil record further shows Australopithecus had molar teeth. Therefore, for the time of emergence of Australopithecus after a period of 58 Ma, his brain was much larger, and his size was much larger, and his intelligence was much more significant in comparison to the first mammals and diet started to shift also to include more different plant food sources and not just fruits and young leaves. At the end of Pliocene (that lasted from two million to 10,000 years ago), weather circumstances started to shift. The Pleistocene was marked by a much colder climate and recurring glaciations of the northern hemisphere. So-called Ice Age. The consequence was that during both epochs, tropical forests shrank and in many areas have disappeared entirely. They were replaced in by savanna woodlands. Tree species decreased, the climate became more seasonal, and primates in the expanding savanna areas must have faced many new dietary challenges. Specialized carnivores and herbivores that thrive in the African savannas were evolving at the same time as early humans competing for scarce food sources of bared savanna landscape. This conditions had to force our ancestors to adapt even more perhaps to become a new type of omnivore, one entirely dependent on social and technological innovation and not just foraging. Thus, forcing adaptation that requires to a great extent increased brainpower.

Edward O. Wilson of Harvard University had done some calculations on expansion of the human brain. The conclusion was that for two million years, brain size grow for about a tablespoon every 100,000 years until the emergence of Homo sapiens, and then the brain growth stopped. The classic line of thought is that the earliest hominins were forced to move from a forested environment to a savanna one and had to adapt by shifting to the harder and tougher food items more common in the new environment. Openness also explains the selective advantages of bipedalism because bipedalism is the most effective form of walking if you are not an arboreal animal. If we look at Australopithecus, he had genuinely massive jaws and molars. The large and thick-enameled teeth of Australopithecines suggest diets that included hard foods. There are only two possible scenarios in that case. It might use its teeth to open strong shells of relatively large seeds. Alternatively, another more plausible scenario is that it used its teeth to focus on starch-rich foods. Many plants have reserved energy in their underground part so-called underground storage organs (USO's), such as bulbs and corms, and it might represent a significant component of Australopithecine diets. The hardness of some raw USO's is sufficient to explain, potentially, the

Australopithecine craniodental morphology. Also, fossils of mole rats that are specialized in eating USO's are found at the same fossil sites with hominins significantly more often than expected by chance. Furthermore, the stable isotope ratio signatures imply that the co-occurring mole rat and hominin fossils may have been consuming similar foods.

Plants carbohydrates serve as energy reserves or for structural functions. Reserve carbohydrates can be stored in different parts of the plant usually seeds and nuts and especially beans can have them to serve as energy for sprouting. Certain fruits have them, and also underground storage organs (USO's) such as tubers, roots, and rhizomes. Edible roots and tubers are very energy dense because they can constitute up to 80% of the dry weight of pure starch. One other advantage is that they remain stable and do not rot if left undisturbed because they are naturally growing in the ground so they can be collected as required across a stretch of time. USO's can also be dried but is questionable if the early hominins had a level of intelligence to apply this technique. Because of the availability and energy density, it has been proposed that USO's have become one of the most essential foods sources for early hominins. Addition of starch-rich USO's was a crucial step in further hominin evolution and expansion into new habitats. USO-rich aquatic habitats such as deltas have been proposed as an intermediate niche in the adaptation of early hominins to savanna habitats. Those two theories (big seeds versus USO's as essential food sources) are not necessarily incompatible. It is very doubtful that any hominin species consumed only one type of food. Some surveys of craniodental morphology suggest significant inter-individual dietary variability even in Australopithecines. What is also important to consider is the possibility that even relatively rarely consumed foods may have been critical for survival in certain periods when preferred foods were not available.

Therefore, fruits, flowers, green leaves and vegetables, USO's and nuts and seeds with no meat, no dairy, no eggs. In hominins from the genus Homo that evolved from Australopithecines, we can see more diversification about 3.5 million years ago. At that time some members also added grasses or sedges to their menus. For another million years that was the diet. The earliest evidence for meat eating in hominins dates to 2.5 Mya. Some of the fossil findings are consistent with scavenging activities with no hunting. Meaning bone marrow or insects or something in similar nature in no more than a couple of percent of overall calories. Something similar to the baboons or chimpanzee's diets. This meat source was insignificant to the scale of producing any physiological adaptation that will translate to any evolutionary change in biology. The adoption of large-scale meat-eating may have necessitated advanced processing techniques, such as cooking, in part because raw meat is full of putrefying bad bacteria and other types of bad micro-organisms and parasites that will eventually kill us if are not killed themselves by a thermal process. Thus limiting consumption in large quantities.

Limiting factor that a large number of scientist do not seem to understand is that meat spoils very quickly in the hot savanna conditions of Africa. In 2h, just two, it is gone. In 15 minutes there would already be insects crawling on top of the carcass and also there would be other predators looking for an easy meal. For example, pack of hyenas. In order to consume meat on a scale that will be significant to create an adaptation, it will have to be the staple of the diet with calorie influx of at least 10 to 15 percent. That will be real omnivorous diet. Without large-scale hunting on a daily basis, that is impossible. Without technology, like traps or spears, it is not a logical assumption and without cooking, it is 100% not liable option.

The earliest authentic proof for human-controlled fire dates to 400,000 years ago in Israel. There are other unproven sites dating to as early as 1.5 Mya. Some scientist suggests that cooking food may have been part of hominin culture as early as 1.9 Mya in this period there was a significant reduction in toot size of Homo erectus. This is only possible if he started to adopt softer diets. This might be because of the use of cooking. Cooking does not just make old food more palatable. It also makes food that was not palatable before, a new source of calories. The real truth is that without baking, many otherwise nutritious tubers would be too tough for consumption. Because of the higher quality diet gut size significantly decreased. This fact just by itself proves the increase in quality of the diet. More calories and lesser digestive tract that used them previously now means more for the brain and size increased even further. There are still vigorous debates about all of this issues. Was cooking the crucial part of developing of a human brain or was its use of Stone Age tools, or whether the adding starch-rich USO's or meat to the diet. What was the most crucial energy source that provided much-needed energy for the development of the brain, you take your own opinion. The debates are emotional in nature, not as logical as science needs to be. It is because of our underlying desire to prove to ourselves that meat consumption is natural for human evolution so that we can justify large scale meat consumption in the modern era. The scientific and archeological data can become a problem in this scenario if data don't reflect the desirable way of looking at things.

The scientists are not immune to emotional bias. In order to have large-scale meat consumption on a daily basis, the two criteria must be met. First one is to have a viable option of acquiring the meat. The second one is to have the physiological ability to digest it. First criteria for humans that are not anatomical hunters and are slow and week and cannot compete with true anatomical hunters is to scavenge for it. That option will not support the calorie requirement and can only be an additional source of calories in small extent. For the second option, we would need to have fire technology. Subsequently anything before Homo erectus is excluded. Some of the scientists believe that even Homo erectus was not capable of controlling the fire. It is a big debate. Notable is that most mammals appear to enjoy the heat radiated at night at sites of recently burned-out fires. Currently, the earliest well-accepted instance of fire-burning in a controlled manner came from Israel's Qesem Cave at 400,000 years ago. However, there is some new research that had been done in South Africa's Wonderwerk Cave. Archaeological excavations there from the 1970s through the 1990s turned up stone hand axes, acheulean tools and different devices that were likely created by Homo erectus. In 2004, the new excavations had been conducted by the team of researchers led by Francesco Berna of Boston University. In the cave, there was ash from burned plants and charred bone fragments. Employing a method named Fourier Transform Infrared Microspectroscopy, the team determined the temperature reach more than 900 degrees Fahrenheit, with, leaves, grasses or brush used as fuel. Creating and controlling fire was a transformative development in the history of humans. Actually for Homo erectus who mastered it. There are also other sites. At Chesowanja, for example, archaeologists found fire-hardened clay fragments, dated to 1.42 Mya. Fire allowed our ancestor to cook and cooked food is already predigested, so it was easier to digest and is providing more calories. At the same time, the hominin gut shrank, freeing up the energy needed to its functioning. The saved energy was then devoted to fueling the evolution of bigger brains. A brain is energetically speaking the most expensive organ to maintain. A brain needs 22 times as many power to operate in the form of spent energy as an equivalent amount of muscle.

If Homo erectus mastered the use of fire as archeological record seems to confirm, the origin of Homo erectus, some 1.9 million years ago should be used as a time of significant transition. H. erectus had smaller faces, smaller teeth, and jaws, larger brains, shorter intestinal tracts. All of this thanks to higher quality diet made by roasting of tubers. H. erectus brain size began to expand, and the hominin body became taller and more modern. Cooking of USO's rich in starch is what influenced our physiology and combined with foraging based on behavioral adaptations fueled even larger brain development. What fire does is that brakes molecular structure of food and in a sense simulate the process of digesting. Therefore, what it does is that it is not just making unusable food digestible but also makes digestible food more nutritious because it frees up the calories in it. Fire makes them more available so we would get more calories from the same food that we had been eating before. Starch is digested slowly and incompletely if it is in raw crystalline form, but more efficiently after cooking. Eating raw potatoes for example is never a good idea.

Cooking starch-rich plant foods coevolved with increased salivary amylase activity in the human lineage. Humans are unusual in that they have very high levels of the salivary α-amylase. In a genetic sense, it is due to multiple copies of AMY1 genes. Among primates, multiple copy numbers of AMY1 genes have been identified only in H. sapiens. Humans have two types of - α amylases, one expressed in salivary glands, and the other is expressed in the pancreas. Salivary amylase begins starch hydrolysis immediately during mastication in the oral cavity. Young infants have minimal pancreatic amylase activity. When nondairy foods are introduced into the diet following weaning, a large part of starch digestion, possibly 50%, is accomplished by salivary amylases.

In contrast in adults, the starch is primarily digested in the duodenum. This appears to be a result of multiple DNA retroviral insertions. First at 43 Mya, then after that, we experienced a second upstream retroviral insertion around 39 Mya. This was a required adaptation because of the shift in the diet that was moving away from predominantly fructose from fruits and fats from nuts and seeds to a more starch-based diet. Rapid growth in hominin brain size during the Middle Pleistocene also required an increased supply of preformed glucose. Cooking starch-rich plant foods pushed this adaptation even further and coevolved with increased salivary amylase activity. Without cooking of starch-rich plant foods that allowed better absorption and allowed us to eat otherwise uneatable plants, it is unlikely that the high demand for calories of modern humans will be met. The regular consumption of energy-dense starchy plant foods gives us a sound solution for the requirement of additional energy source to explain growing brain during the Late Pliocene and Early Pleistocene. Most of the people that are not familiar with this science somehow developed the baseline of thinking that modern humans discovered fire in the Stone Age and that increased brain size of modern humans is a consequence of meat eating in our hominin ancestors. Reality is that Homo erectus discovered fire and that cooking starches and a hard time thinking for optimal foraging solutions give rise to our intelligence.

Roasting USO's is what made us human not bone marrow. And no there is no need to go entirely raw that is not a human diet, it is primate diet and hominin diet before Homo erectus. Optimal human diet can be from 30 to 60 percent raw. Cooking is literally what made us human. Well at least that 0.5 to 1 percent in the genetic difference between H. erectus and us.

Now for the first option of acquiring the meat on a sustainable basis, we will have to have a way of killing a pray that is fast and conditioned to be chased by fast predators. In other words, we will have to have some traps or spears. The first hominin who could have done this is theoretically Homo erectus. Problem with this is that we do not see any evidence of technology except fire and stone tools. There are some scientists that have a thesis that Homo erectus used fire to bate, isolate and kill the animals, but in that scenario, he would have to had much higher intelligence. Using fire for hunting is not using fire, it is using wildfire. Wildfire can spread into large areas and can devastate the habitat and plant food sources and can burn the Homo erectus himself and his cave and half of Africa. If we assume that he was so smart to control the use of wildfire, something even modern firefighters have a problem with, we will have to level the Homo erectus intelligence to a greater extent. If he was capable of doing this, then he would be capable of creating other technologies like traps. That would allow him to spread to cold climates with snow and ice and that was not the case.

Stone tools and animal bone debris does not mean sustainable hunting on a large scale and real meat infused omnivorous diet. It means scavenging some meat left behind by big predators if we are lucky and crack opening the bones and head to eat the brain and bone marrow and occasionally killing some of the young and defenseless animals or injured or something in that nature. All of this can happen but on some lucky special occasions and not on large scale daily hunting as Neanderthals did. Complex trapping methods to entrap and kill antelopes, gazelles, wild beast and other large animals let me repeat this is not posable without weapons. If I jump on a gazelle, there would be two options. Gazelle will just run off or kicked me in the gut first and then run off. When we look at human hunting, it always relays on traps, bows, and arrows or other weapons to kill or spear to injure and then persistence hunting until the antelope is exhausted. All methods require the use of technology. Persistence hunting just by itself is not enough because that would mean running for tens of miles for pray and then carrying that pray for tens of miles and if we are lucky not to been seen by another big predator and became meal ourselves. Even if this is posable carrots tend to run slower than the rabbits so if there are plant sources around hunting is not an option if we understand the optimal foraging strategies. Problem is logical because as soon this is acquired, guess what, that species can spread to cooler climate without abundant plant food sources.

The first hominin to have both conditions wright was the Neanderthal and he spread to ice could Europe before us where he hunted large pray. Also, one other thing, even him did not like it. Nobody likes to hunt. We have this kind of romantic view of hunting where we think it is the macho manly thing that we enjoy like we enjoy playing video games. The truth is that it is a most dangerous life-threatening process that exists in nature not just to pray but for a hunter too. If not successful there is a lot of energy loss, and even if it is successful with no injuries, there will be a lot of pain and exhaustion. In the Ice Age in Europe going through five feet of snow is not easy, and there are cold temperatures, and we can die from cold or slip and fall and hit our had or twist an ankle or break bones or fall into icy water. In summer or in Africa, we could get bitten by a poisonous snake or get in contact with the poisonous plant or fall in quicksand in the swamp or just get attacked by a wild pack of lions or hyenas or get stung by a swarm of wild bees. That means if we were lucky and didn't get into the territory of another hominin. Nature at that time was the dangerous and wild place. If a modern man that knows how to survive in nature with all of our technology lose himself in wilderness, the possibility for survival in an extended period is zero. In the wild nature of the past possibilities for death are endless. Hunting for hominins and humans are an extreme tactic for survival if nothing else is available. In another hand, if we are foraging and stumble upon a fresh corps of some animal half eaten, well lucky us.

Consumption of animal products was insignificant in a scale of forcing adaptation of hominin and human physiology. Our natural diet was based on fruits, flowers, leaves and in later times vegetables and of USO-s, nuts and seeds and grains. In more recent times (1 Ma) after the invention of cooking, we have eaten grains, legumes and other more difficult to digest USO's and meat consumption was a couple of percent of total calories. First real omnivores where Neanderthals to some extent, not humans. We did not evolve in Europe we came out of Africa and entered Europe and other cold places around a hundred thousand years ago. That is an insignificant time in evolution.

Moreover, even Neanderthals did not like it and were extremely mall adapted to it. They were forced to do it to survive. The stereotypical representation of Neanderthals pictures them as killing the woolly mammoth. There is archeological evidence to back up a thesis of Neanderthal carnivorous diet even at the same level of the polar bears, that included meals heavy in large herbivores like the woolly mammoth, reindeer and woolly rhinoceros. However, Neanderthal teeth tell a different story. Dental plaque is used to analyze the starches and proteins that were preserved in the plaque. When investigated the wear patterns on their teeth suggest a varied diet. Diet also varied depending on a location with significant regional differences. In some areas studies imply that Neanderthals were consuming mostly plants, possibly including medicinal ones.

The significant discovery came when scientist analyzed the remains of Neanderthals from El Sidrón, Spain. The Neanderthals from El Sidrón showed zero signs of meat consumption. Not some small amount but complete round zero. Instead of meat, they got calories from plant foods gathered from the forest. Dental plaque was filled with remains of different kinds of nuts, mushrooms, and moss. Neanderthal vegans, how could that fit in the typical accepted image? What about protein and b12? Dental plaque is a very useful tool because it can preserve genetic material from the food that animals eat for analysis. Laura Weyrich at the University of Adelaide and a team of researchers were able to produce an amazingly accurate look at what plant and animal species Neanderthals had been eating. They analyzed three samples. Two obtained fossils were from El Sidrón Cave in Spain, including the potential aspirin-popper, while one was from Spy Cave in Belgium. The analysis again proved the complete diversity of food depending on local habitat ecology that was in the line of optimal foraging theory (OFT). Neanderthal diet didn't exist in essence. Diet depended on where the Neanderthals in question lived. The Belgians, for example, followed the meat-heavy pattern because they had to. Genetic material from wild sheep, woolly rhinoceros, and some mushrooms was discovered in dental plaque with also some bones in the cave from horses, mammoth, reindeer, and rhinoceros. Bones tell the identical story as the dental plaque that these groups were hunters. In Belgian habitat, they did not forage for plant foods because there wasn't any to be found. They had to adapt to survive cold barren climate by hunting. They probably didn't like it too much either.

The Spanish Neanderthals appeared to have a more comfortable life. They eat largely mushrooms, pine nuts, and moss and other kinds of food we would get from foraging in a forest. Thus Neanderthals from the north were hunters, Neanderthals from the south were foragers. What this evidence tell us? One of the Neanderthals from Spain appeared to have a dental abscess and stomach bug and was self-medicating with poplar (Populus alba), a natural painkiller containing salicylic acid, the same active ingredient in the aspirin. The individual had also consumed the antibiotic-producing mold Penicillium. That is tens of thousands of years before Dr. Alexander Fleming used a strain of Penicillium to develop the first antibiotic, revolutionizing modern medicine. If we want to talk about founders of medicine, well how about antibiotic and aspirin popping Neanderthals. One another thing was interesting. Weyrich's team also managed to completely sequence one particular microbe called Methanobrevibacter oralis that lacks genes for resisting antiseptics and digesting maltose. In time this microbe has adapted to hygiene and changing human diets. Weyrich's team calculated that the Neanderthal strain split apart from those found in modern humans between 112,000 and 143,000 years ago which suggests that the two groups were trading Methanobrevibacter likely when they had sex.

So why are groups of Neanderthals living in the south being vegan? Probably because they can. There were in much more friendly surrounding and milder climate with more food sources. If we have something we can eat growing beside our cave would we go to hunt? Just applying optimal foraging strategies, we have the answer. Neanderthals were anatomically more vegan then carnivorous, but in the northern parts during Ice Age, the climate was harsh and they had to adapt and that took some time. Both Neanderthals and modern humans evolved from Homo erectus. The earliest known migration waves of H. erectus into Eurasia dated to 1.81 million years ago. Molecular clock genetic research had placed the divergence time of the Neanderthal and modern human lineages from 800,000 to 400,000 years ago. For this reason, most scholars believe Neanderthals descend, via Homo heidelbergensis. Homo erectus population that stayed in Africa would have evolved through the intermediate Homo rhodesiensis, into anatomically modern humans by 300,000 years ago or earlier.

Neanderthal evolved in Europe and humans did in Africa and there are some small physiological differences. Homo sapiens have smaller barrel-shaped chests and narrow pelvises. Neanderthals had bell-shaped torsos with wider pelvises. The conventional explanation has been that Neanderthals needed more oxygen due to the colder climate, so their bodies grew to hold a bigger respiratory system. But this is wrong. Living in the cold climate of Eurasia 300,000 to 30,000 years ago, Neanderthals settled in places like the Polar Urals and southern Siberia. In the midst of a tundra winter, with no plant food sources to be found, animal meat made of fat and protein remained the only energy source. Although the fat is easier to digest, it is scarce in cold conditions. Prey animals burned up their fat stores during the winter and became much leaner. The conclusion must be made that Neanderthals must have been eating a great deal of animal protein. Protein places huge requirements on kidneys and liver to remove some of the toxic byproducts produced by burning it for energy. Humans have a protein ceiling of between 35 and 50 percent of calories in our diet. Eating much more than that can be dangerous. Neanderthals bodies found a way to utilize more protein by enlarging liver and kidneys. Chests and pelvises widened also to accommodate these beefed-up organs giving them distinct look. If we look today at Inuit peoples, their diet subsists at times on all-meat and nothing else and they do have larger livers and kidneys and longer ribs than average Europeans. To survive the fat famine, Neanderthals undoubtedly also specialized in hunting massive animals like mammoths. They retain fat longer in poor conditions and require less energy and speed to kill than smaller swifter pray. Mammoths are too big to escape or evade, and we only have to kill one to feast for months because meat does not spoil in constant subzero temperatures. But as these mega-beasts vanished, Neanderthals likely struggled to chase down smaller, swifter prey. In the southern part like Spain, they went old vegan way. What all of this tells us about us. We didn't have over the millennia of living in Ice Age northern climate to adapt to a diet rich in meat to some extent. We evolved in Africa from plan based vegan lineage of 60 million years. Modern humans first left Africa 100,000 years ago in a series of slow-paced migration waves and arrived in southern Europe around 80,000-90,000 years ago. Therefore, what is the real paleo diet?

Homo sapiens dietary evolution

"Tell me what you eat, and I will tell you what you are." - Jean Anthelme Brillat-Savarin

Human diet can be a lot of different things in a lot of different environments. We are classified as omnivorous species. We can be vegan or Inuit Eskimos, and we will still survive. Finding food in almost every environment is what make us adaptable and made as spread across the world but we use technology, and our bodies evolved in the time period counting in millions of years so the big question emerges: What are we adapted at eating, not what we can eat? We can eat anything even other humans, and we will live but what is optimal diet for us that will sustain us without any complications? Our current form of Homo sapiens emerged 300,000 years ago. From that time until now we are the same. Somehow most people have trouble with this. Yes, we are the same. If we take a human from 250,000 years ago and put him in the current world, he would finish college, get married, had kids, and you would not know that he had traveled through time. He would have no apparent differences at all.

Now to be precise there were some adaptations that happened. In the same way, some of the similar adaptations existed in Neanderthals too but they happened in humans separately. We did not inherit them from our Neanderthal cousins. In new environmental conditions they emerged independently. One of them, for example, is paling of the skin caused by systematic vitamin D deficiency. Other more modern, just human thing would be for example lactose tolerance in European populations. People from European descent can drink milk and rest of the globe cannot. Black Africans are 98 percent lactose intolerant and numbers in Asia are similar. When we start to do something unnatural to our bodies, in time we will adapt to it in some way, but if we change the way we live to rapidly we are a done deal.

Moreover, that is precisely what the Industrial Revolution did. The Neolithic revolution did it to a smaller extent, but Industrial Revolution devastated our natural life and order. What will happen if sub-Saharan Africans drink milk? There were cases of deaths when smart people from the UN were sending powdered milk as humanitarian aid and that milk ended up in the chronically malnourished children meals. To some extent, we are that African child maladapted to our modern life and diet, and we are poisoned chronically because of the maladaptations. Our natural state is not to be hunchback fat chronically diseased dying pill popping unhappy addicts.

Food is not just food. Food is combination of millions of different chemicals that affect our genes and biological system. We are what we eat. So what are we designed to eat? The short answer would be the same thing that Homo erectus had been eating, but the longer answer would be that we are omnivores and that we could potentially thrive on a much-diversified diet then that of our hominin ancestor. However, what precisely that definition means. Chimpanzees, for example, are classified as omnivores because they can find and eat a termite from time to time. So what? Importance of that food source is limited because rest of the time 98 percent of calories would come from regular and more available plant sources and that meat source would not be able to create any form of meaningful evolutional adaptation in their internal organs or constitution, but they are still classified as omnivores. In veterinary school they learn that cats are carnivores; rabbits, horses, and ruminants are herbivores; and dogs and pigs like people are omnivores. However, how can that be? Wolves also eat grains. It is said that not only will they indulge themselves to some occasional berries, but also they will eat grains contained in the stomach of their prey. Lately, it has been found that dogs are distinctive from their wild cousins as they have three genes related to the digestion of starch and glucose. This would be a form of evolutional adaptation that happened in the period from the first domestication. As such, it is hard to deny that dogs are specially adapted at eating grains and other vegetation. However, at this point we could have a problem.

If chimpanzees are omnivores and dogs are omnivores would that mean that their physiology must be similar? In certain conditions when there is an absolute need, the herbivorous animals will eat available meat only to survive. The deer will, for example, begin to chew on fresh carrion when he is deficient in certain nutrients. For instance, calcium can be obtained by chewing bone. Also, many of the seemingly herbivorous animals may hunt for meat sometimes. There are videos on YouTube where a panda is seen hunting a peacock, killing it and eating it afterward. The reason why they do this may be caused by the hunger, or the peacock somehow triggered their ancestral hunting instinct. Nevertheless, it proves that even herbivores are not absolute herbivores. Moreover, the reverse is also true, where known carnivores would also eat grass to a lesser degree. We will have to look at this in more detail. Problem with this analysis can arise in the form of psychological issues that can move us away from the real scientific analysis. It is what I like to call "we are the omnivores" argument that serves as the point of justification in the conscious mind based on subconscious desire for supernormal stimuli of food gratification. In real life scientific view, it is problematic too because omnivores diet is a gray area. Biochemistry does not work in gray areas. The liver creates cholesterol or it doesn't. It is not possible to one-day secrete cholesterol in the bloodstream but on another day when we eat a steak, somehow our bodies will sense that external dietary cholesterol is there in the bloodstream in order to stop production for that day. Biochemistry does not function in that way, and I will say unfortunately for us. Our bodies will try to remove excess cholesterol trough colon by injecting it into the digestive system with a hope that if would bind to the fiber and leave. And that is all our bodies can do. If you don't eat enough fiber it will just get reabsorbed back. In carnivore species, their livers do not create any cholesterol because they get it with every bite. For meat eaters cholesterol is an essential nutrient. For us, it is not. Usually, people do not understand this. No matter how much cholesterol carnivores eat they do not develop atherosclerosis. When plant eaters eat their plants, they do not get it, and their liver produces it. However, when plant eaters for millions of years suddenly begin to eat excessive amounts of dietary cholesterol then the heart attack follows. In respect of the biochemistry of cholesterol production, we can have only carnivorous and herbivorous. No gray area in there. Also, we can have dogs that don't create cholesterol and are omnivorous but still get most of their calorie needs from meat, and we can have chimps that are omnivorous but get 98 percent from plant foods. Essentially what we have is an omnivorous dog from carnivorous descent and omnivorous chimp from herbivorous descent but in almost every physiological way chimp is plant eater, and the dog is a meat eater. So what about us? Our livers do create cholesterol, so we are omnivorous of heart attack descent. Paleo people who like their lean meat somehow forget that in the paleo period most prehistoric peoples did not live long enough to die from cardiovascular disease. In extreme harsh conditions where average life expectancy is 32 years of age, the genes that get passed along to younger generations are the ones that are just old enough to go to reproductive age by any means necessary. That means not dying of starvation or disease or in an attack. The more calories we consume, the better no matter what they are. Eating whatever we can find including bone marrow on special occasions or even human meat would have a selective advantage. Think of it in this way. If we only have to live long enough to get to pass along our genes and to protect our kids until puberty, would you care about the heart attack? We can have a good example if we look at vitamin C too. For meat eaters, vitamin C is not a vitamin. Because vitamin C is only found in plant kingdom meat eaters produce their own. For species that are plant eaters, vitamin C is a vitamin. It is a necessary nutrient that we must consume, or we die. In the Middle Ages, sailors died from scurvy on a regular basis. They did not know what that disease was for a long period of time. It was in 1614, when John Woodall, Surgeon General of the East India Company, published "The Surgeon's Mate" as a handbook for apprentice surgeons aboard the company's ships. What he noted in the book was already established knowledge from decades of experience of mariners that have accidentally found out that the scurvy can be treated with fresh food or, if not available, limes, oranges, lemons, and tamarinds. He was, regardless, unable to clarify the science behind all of this, and his statement that scurvy was a digestive disease had no real effect on the opinions of the influential physicians who ran the medical establishment at that time. True omnivores like bears do not die from scurvy. The reason why Eskimos did not suffer from vitamin C deficiency is because they eat nothing but the raw meat and livers of animals they catch. Vitamin C is sensitive to heating, so when we use fire or cooking, meat loses even the small amount that was in it, but then the unprocessed meat is a death sentence for any humans that lived outside of the polar circle because of our low resistance filter.

Carnivorous species deal with bad microorganisms with strong stomach acid. The capacity of the carnivore stomach to emit hydrochloric acid is outstanding. Carnivores can hold their gastric pH all way down to around 1 or 2, even with food present. Strong gastric pH facilitates protein breakdown and is necessary to kill the abundant amount of dangerous microorganisms frequently found in rotting flesh. When we eat a rotten apple, we might get drunk, but if we eat raw decaying flesh, there is an excellent possibility for severe consequences and death. Eating raw meat from decaying carcasses is not our food. For instance, vultures stomach acid is particularly corrosive, enabling them to safely digest rotten meat tainted with hog cholera bacteria, botulinum toxin and anthrax bacteria that would be deadly even to other scavengers. New World vultures often vomit when threatened or approached. High levels of stomach acidity developed not only to help animals break down food but more importantly to defend animals against food poisoning. The bacteria that will putrefy the fruit, for example, will do nothing to meat. It is a different kind of bacteria. Gastric acidity is one of the critical factors in the determination of microbiome composition (microbial communities found in the gut). Species feeding on carrion require the strongest stomach acidity possible as protection from foreign microbes. Herbivores on another hand should require lower restrictive filter, as the risk of infection is lower. To cope with the increased risk of a wide range of pathogens the carnivores and all other animals that eat meat like scavengers and omnivores have developed significantly higher stomach acidities. If we compare the acidity of the average scavenger with an acidity of an average grazer, we can see that stomach acid acts as a biological filter. When species with low stomach acid consume even fresh raw meat, the defensive mechanism is significantly lowered because low acidity and food poisoning is a concern. Stomach acidity of carnivores is around pH 1 with food in the stomach. True omnivore also has the acidity of pH 1 with food in the stomach. With humans and also other herbivores acidity is around pH 4 to 5 with food in the stomach. Just this fact alone tells a lot about what we are. Never eat raw animal products. Never. No raw eggs no raw milk no raw nothing. If it is from animal and it is raw, then it is not our food. Even heating sometimes cannot kill all the nasty microorganisms that live in meat.

You probably heard the term pasteurization. Pasteurization is the reason for milk's extended shelf life. It is named after the French scientist Louis Pasteur. When he heated wine, he discovered that it would not go bad and that heating it was enough to stop spoilage. He found the way to prevent beverages from going sour. Beverage contamination also led Pasteur to the idea that micro-organisms are infecting animals and humans and are able to cause disease in the same way that they spoil the wine leading Joseph Lister to develop antiseptic methods in surgery. Before massive population expansion and urban growth caused by industrialization people kept dairy cows even in the cities. The reason was to shorten the period between production and consumption in order to minimize the disease risk associated with ingestion of raw milk. For example, between 1912 and 1937 there were around 65,000 reported deaths caused by tuberculosis contracted from contaminated milk in England and Wales alone.

Today all food products that can cause disease by carrying some form of germs must be pasteurized mandatory including fruit juices. Pasteurization also kills more than just bacteria it kills most of the nutrients that are not thermostable. Entire debate of row against cooked food is raging because of this. Because we are not true omnivores that are designed to digest raw animal products all of this is absolutely necessary, and I will repeat it never eat raw eggs or milk or meat. Even raw vegetables that have been contaminated by human or animal feces can carry them, therefore washing is necessary and homegrown sprouting for salads is not recommended. There are also parasites that can live in the flesh, not just bacteria. Stomach acid of true omnivores and carnivores would be enough to kill all of these parasites, but ours is not. Today in modern medicine the treatment is available for most of the foodborne parasitic organisms but not for all of them. One more issue we need to mention here. Pasteurization is not the same as Sterilization. The sterilization process kills all forms of microbial life, including spores, fungi, viruses, and bacteria. Sterilization is performed using different strategies, for example by applying heat, irradiation, chemicals and applying high pressure. Sterilization allows us to store food and liquids for prolonged periods; however, it can also reduce any helpful bacteria that may be present in food as well. Furthermore, the procedure also changes the taste of the food. Sterilization is also used in the medical field to prevent bacteria or viruses from spreading and causing infections. For instance, all equipment needs to be sterilized before a patient goes to operation.

In regular cooking pasteurization is fine. Some microbes can survive pasteurization. Bacteria and yeasts can sporulate. Spores are hard to kill; they are almost alien creatures that are very resistant. It will take the high temperature for an extended period to kill them. When the bacteria or yeasts are starving or sense a change in the environment, like extreme temperatures and drought, they will produce a spore. This spore is a form of a protective outer layer that is remarkably resilient and protective. It can help the germ survive for decades by living in the form of a dormant state. It is still not clear how the cell survives without nutrition in these conditions. Once environmental conditions improve, the spore will break. If by some accident you get yourself locked up and want to drink some hooch all you need is a slice of old bread and some sugary base like juice. Yeast spores in bread would do the rest. People who have yeast triggered immune system reactions like Chron's disease and candida overgrowth should avoid eating bread, and anything else made with yeast even if it is baked or cooked. However, for most of the time pasteurization is just fine and most of the microorganisms will be killed at 161 F or 71 C in 16 seconds. Except for heat-resistant spores. All spores will be killed by sterilization at 121 C for 15 min.

The reason we get a fever is to stop the multiplication of microorganisms. Fever will not be high enough to kill them directly because it would mean killing our cells too. Rising body temperature will only harden the division and multiplying until the immune system kicks them off. In my mind, we should never take aspirin or anything else to lower the fever if it is not absolutely necessary. It will just make a recovery longer and more difficult.

Another problem for us is not just low acidity; it is also the shape and length of our intestines. Due to the relative difficulty with which various types of plant foods are broken down (due to large amounts of non-digestible fibers), herbivores have longer intestines than carnivores significantly. The human intestine is long and coiled, just like that of cows, horses, and apes. Long intestines make the digestion process slow and the reason why is to allow adequate time for complete absorption of all nutrients. The small intestine in all herbivore animals tends to be very long, greater than ten times body length. Grazers, for example, need two chamber stomachs to ferment a high proportion of cellulose. Herbivores that eat relatively soft vegetation do not need a multi-chambered stomach. They usually have a simple stomach and a long small intestine. These animals ferment the hard-to-digest fibrous parts of their diets in their colon.

In contrast, the intestine of a carnivore is short, straight and tubular. Because meat is relatively easily digested, there is no fiber in meat, remains can be excreted quickly before they start to rot. Their small intestines are short about three to five times the length of their body. Many of herbivores increase the efficiency of their GI tracts by including enzymes that digest carbohydrates in their saliva. Human saliva contains the digestive enzyme for carbohydrates, salivary amylase. This enzyme is essential for the absorption of starch. The reason we chew is not just to grind the fiber but also because we need to infuse the food with digestive enzymes. The esophagus is narrow. Large chunks of meat and bone will not be able to go through. Carnivores do not produce enzymes in salivary glands and therefore don't need to chew on the meat and sometimes when pray is small enough they would swallow the whole thing. Because of the difference in time needed to fully absorb nutrients from fiber rich foods and the length of the intestine the transit time (time needed for food to go through whole digestive system from mouth to the anus) between humans and carnivores is what really brings all of the anatomical differences back home. In the 1980s, Mayo Clinic researchers measured digestion time in 21 healthy people. Total transit time, from eating to elimination in the stool, averaged 53 hours. Let repeat this again, 53 hours. Average transit time in a pure carnivore such as the mink, for example, is 2.4 hours! The difference exists because the transit time of our colon is 30 to 40 hours. Just colon by itself. After leaving the stomach and small intestine food has to be fermented in colon and carnivores do not need this because meat is easily digested because it does not contain fiber. All of the fats and proteins can be extracted in the small intestine, and colon has no purpose. This then means that when people eat meat, it has plenty of time to putrefy and cause the production of cancer-causing agents. Because we do not have acid that is strong enough to sterilize meat some of the nasty germs can survive, consequently death from food poisoning is guaranteed if raw (spoiled) meat is consumed on a regular basis.

The average time for the meat to spoil in a climate of Africa is 2 hours. Butchers recommend getting game down to 40 degrees within an hour of killing. Decay starts immediately, the same second the animal is dead. It can be only slowed by refrigeration. Usually, after killing a deer, the hunter field dresses the animal. That means he cuts the deer open so that he could take the guts out. Guts are filled with bacteria. Next step is to cool down the meat as soon as possible by packing the cavity with ice or snow. The time between a commercially grown animal is slaughtered, butchered, shipped to store, stocked, purchased, put in a fridge, then taken out to cook can be quite a while. For most of that time, the meat must be cold but still will accumulate microbes. When it hits room temperature, immediately microorganisms inside start to grow. The idea that somehow Homo erectus with his low acid digestive tract can sustainably eat raw meat carcasses in a climate of Africa is idiotic, and the idea that he had been able to hunt down and then control fire to roast the meat would elevate his intelligence to the level of modern humans and that is not the case. Leading causes of hospitalization caused by foodborne illness in the US is Salmonella with 35% followed by norovirus 26%, and the leading causes of death caused by foodborne illness are also salmonella with 28%. When we look at E.coli levels of contamination in meat which is an indicator of fecal matter contamination, around 70% of beef is contaminated and around 80% of poultry. Why are we buying this contaminated meat? In 1974 American Publick Health Association sued the USDA for approving meat contaminated with Salmonella, you know that lovely stamp that you can see and think it is all ok and safe not realizing the industry is corrupt. The USDA pointed out that: "There have been Salmonella outbreaks linked to dairy and eggs too and that since there are numerous sources of contamination, it would be unjustified to single out the meat industry and ask that the Department require labeling its products as hazardous to health."

This is beyond idiotic, it is almost laughable. In other words, they do not care if your child dies they wont to make many mullahs and they have a corrupt system to protect them. The DC Circuit Court of Appeals upheld the meat industry position because: "American housewives are not normally stupid, and methods of cooking of food do not ordinarily result in food poisoning." Therefore, to recap, selling Salmonella-tainted chicken is legal and has a cute stamp on top of it. Other pathogens in meat include Yersinia enterocolitica in pork, Staphylococcus, MRSA hepatitis E, bladder-infecting E. coli, Clostridium difficile, Campylobacter. In the US about 1 in 7 retail packages of poultry has the Salmonella. Even if we beat it this fecal pathogen can trigger something called Reiter's syndrome. Salmonela can trigger an autoimmune reaction in some cases when you come down with Salmonela food poisoning once and end up with chronic, debilitating arthritis for the rest of your life. Campylobacter is a fecal pathogen that can trigger something called Guillain-Barré syndrome. It is a syndrome where you come down with campylobacter food poisoning once, and end up paralyzed on a ventilator. You are not in a coma, you are awake, but you cannot even breathe on your own. About 50% of European poultry has it, more than 60% in the U.S. But after cooking temperature does what our low acid cannot and kills all of the pathogens. But wait, who undercooks meat?

One thing also to be mentioned is cross contamination. Bacteria on the surface of chicken meat can stick to the chef's knife and hands and can spread into the kitchen environment and subsequently contaminate ready-to-eat foods. We can take meat out of the package, cut it with the knife. Then use the same knife to cut tomatoes for salad and use our hand to cut the bread or already cooked foods. Most people who eat meat are exposed to a small extent to this pathogens true cross-contamination, but immune system kicks them off. With children and with people with low immune status even cross-contamination can be a problem that can get out of control. The reason we do not see this information on the label about cross contamination and potential for existing pathogens in products just advice for safe cooking is because of the industry. They have surveys that show: "That this sort of naming and blaming infection risks to poultry meat and eggs may result in a drop of poultry meat and egg consumption."

What happens is that because there is no warning on the label and there is a stamp of approval people who do not do the research themselves believe in government and system and think that meat is pure and approved, so they do not take precautions. It has the stamp of approval so what is a big problem. Also, what usually happens is that they undercook. Because much of the meat is infected problem can emerge if our immune system became overburden with some other issue. For example, we are overstressed and had flu, and we eat some lovely pink in the middle barbeque, we can get some of the symptoms like diarrhea pain and so on. In the worst case, we can end up in the hospital, and most of us will end up in the hospital sometime in our life due to the food poisoning. More commonly it happens in restaurants with undercooked meat. Especially in the fast food ones. Not all chefs care about food poisoning especially if they have many orders pending. I had worked in the restaurant as a chef, and in the fancy one, not a street joint and I do not write this just like that. If you eat in restaurants, take extra precaution. If you think about this issue, some companies knowingly sell salmonella infected poultry, and they do not want it on the label. Consequently, they knowingly accept the fact that some of the consumers not knowing that meat is infected, will undercook it, and possibly end up in a hospital or worse. And thousands of people every year do die precisely because of this. And we did not even start to count all the parasites, all the drug residues from drugs given to animals to promote growth like for example Ractopamine (muscle growth promoter banned in 160 countries) or just regular drugs and hormones. Also, this is just meat. We can add leukemia viruses in milk to the list and so on, maybe some bird flu.

Bovine leukemia virus (BLV) is a retrovirus which causes enzootic bovine leukosis in cattle. It is frequently found in milk around 80% of milk has it and it is a leading cancer killer in cattle. At a big factory farm 100 %, all of the milk is infected. BLV-infected cells cause B cell leukosis in 1-5% of infected cattle. The reason more cattle do not die from tumors is that they are slaughtered as soon as ready. BLV is closely related to the human T-lymphotropic virus type 1 (HTLV-I). In 1976 it was discovered that BLV could infect the human, chimpanzee and monkey cells. Chimps infants fed with BLV milk developed leukemia and died, and chimps never have leukemia normally. In the decade following the discovery of BLV, studies failed to find antibodies against BLV in humans that led to the prevailing view that human exposure to BLV is not significant and, therefore, the virus is not a public health risk. However, back in 2003 in this research (AIDS Res Hum Retroviruses. 2003 Dec;19(12):1105-13.) they reviewed this issue using more sensitive immunological techniques available today. Using immunoblotting to analyze sera from 257 humans for the four-isotype antibodies (IgA, IgM, IgG1, and IgG4) to the BLV capsid antigen (p24), at least one isotype of reactive BLV antibody was detected in 74% of the sera human tested. The results do not necessarily mean that humans are infected with BLV; the antibodies could be a response to dead BLV we consumed in food it does not mean we were actively infected with the virus. To prove infection, we will have to find the retrovirus actively stitched into our DNA.

In 2014, in published findings in the CDC's Emerging Infectious Diseases journal they did that. They analyze the tissue of breast cancer patients surgeries and 44% of samples tested positive. In subsequent studies, the presence of bovine leukemia virus DNA in breast tissues was strongly associated with diagnosed and confirmed breast cancer. It was estimated that up to 37% of breast cancer cases might be attributable to exposure to BLV and this is just one type of cancer that had been tested!

Next time you want to eat that lovely pink in the middle burger, don't. It is an excellent example of what one maladaptation in an evolutionary sense can do like inadequate acidity to digest meat. If we had stomach acidity of regular hyena, we might get away with large-scale industrial meat production. The acidity of ph1 is enough not only to dissolve bones but a metal penny too. Because we do not, then maladaptation can cause ripple effects like the never-ending story. So how does the industry deal with all of this? We have to understand that large-scale meat production factory stile is not natural. It is not natural to torture the animals in gestation crates. It is not a healthy environment for the animals. You might don't care, but in nature, there is no free meal. Unnatural conditions cause unnatural states. In this situation where animals are crowded one on top of the other, it is a breeding ground for pathogens. Therefore, what will industry going to do to deal with this situation? Any ideas? Well, we can give them antibiotics from day one and case closed …well not just yet.

Have you ever heard of antibiotic resistant Salmonella? If you did you would probably already be dead. Most of the antibiotics produced are not for humans. In America more than 80 percent of all antibiotics are used in meat and poultry production. It is one situation when we use antibiotics occasionally when we are sick, but completely different story when some animals are continuously on them. Than the offspring is always on them and so on. They have to be because of unnaturally crowded conditions they are forced to be in industrialized operations. If there are antibiotics that are constantly present in environment, advantageous mutations can also be transferred through the exchange of plasmids within the entire bacterial colony, leading to a proliferation of resistance. The high animal density in the small space in modern industrial farming results in the sharing of both commensal flora and pathogens, which may favor a rapid spread of infectious agents. Due to usual genetic deviations in bacterial populations, individual bacteria may carry mutations that will make antibiotics less effective. In time this will give a survival advantage to the mutated strain.

Another big problem is that advantageous mutations can also be transferred via plasmid exchange within the bacterial colony anywhere in the world not just on the farm, resulting in a proliferation of the resistance trait. In prolonged periods, this practice is not sustainable because of the process of evolutionary selection. Eventually most of the bacteria will be resistant to some extent. That will accelerate the use of more aggressive antibiotics, and the cycle will continue until more aggressive strains emerge, and animals start to die, and some germ mutates even more, and we all die. This is not over exaggeration, if nothing were changed we would all go back to the Middle Ages. Even the simple routine operations or infections can become death hazard without antibiotics. Just in the United States alone, more than 2 million people are diagnosed with antibiotic-resistant infections. Each year around 23,000 people dies due to antibiotic-resistant infections (CDC). In 2013, the CDC published a report on antibiotic resistance and classified the first 18 species of resistant bacteria as urgent, dangerous or problematic threats.

This was the reason why policies have changed. Sub-therapeutic doses in animal feed have been eliminated as of January 1, 2017, following the new FDA directive. This method has been outlawed in Europe since 2006. They have known about this practices from the beginning, and that is a long time. In the 1950s, a group of US scientists discovered that adding antibiotics to animal feed increases the growth rate of livestock. Not until we created mutated strains and thousands of people start to die every year they did anything. That is the industry way. World Organization for Animal Health, now say that: "Without antibiotics, there would be supply problems of animal protein for the human population." What would we do now without animal protein? We pushed the manipulation of natural laws to literally brink of extinction creating supergerm mutants, but we like and can't go without our animal protein. Supergerms can likewise expand beyond the farm and hospitals and threaten public health through environmental transmission and have the possibility to alter ecosystem balance. This can happen in several different ways, particularly by manure applied to fields as fertilizer or farm runoff or by workers. If antibiotic-resistant microorganism spread outside of the farm, they can transfer their resistant genes to other genera of species, not just other bacteria, that have never been anywhere near antibiotics.

This can happen in lakes, in wild animals, and even in the human digestive tract altering our microbiome. A one published study that analyzed the South Platte River have found that in river sediments downstream from more massive feedlots (ones with 10,000 cattle) antibiotic resistance genes were 10,000 times higher compared to river sediment upstream from such feedlots. To deal with pathogens without antibiotics industry pushed FDA and now it has been approved by FDA a mixture of live viruses, bacteria-eating viruses to be precise, as a meat additive. What they intend to do is to use live viruses in processing plants for spraying onto ready-to-eat meat or to fed the viruses to the animals directly as a fed. Viruses were isolated from poultry carcasses. There is no danger to humans because viruses only attack bacteria and therefore they can be used to reduce colonization in the live birds and would not introduce any new biological entity into the food chain. In other words, we already eat them in a small amount. They are on the meat to begin with, so consumers should not complain. They are only being used for Listeria so far. Listeria is a type of foodborne bacteria with rare ability to survive in an acidic, cold, salty environment, in other words, known as hot dogs, deli meats, and refrigerated, ready-to-eat chicken and turkey products. The mortality rate of infection with Listeria is 20 to 30%, making it the number one most dangerous microorganism in the meat supply.

The funny fact about it all is that we cannot even taste the meat itself. We do not have amino acid receptors in our tongue. Only for one. It is so called the fifth taste. The receptor is reactive to the amino acid glutamate, aka umami. Industry loves it because the can put glutamate aka MSG into anything and make it taste like an explosion. Carnivorous animals do taste all of the aminos in their mouths. We can taste fat and texture of meat and salt and spices but licking raw meat is tasteless. In comparison, if we give the cat a pure sugar, it would not taste it at all. It would be like water. Carnivorous animals do not have receptors for glucose in their tongue, but when they lick blood or meat, it is the same as us licking the sugar. Somehow I find that most people have even hard time accepting this, so here is one study: Cats Lack a Sweet Taste Receptor; doi: 10.1093/jn/136.7.1932S.

Jaws are different too. Herbivores have jaws that can go in any direction. Carnivorous animals or true omnivores that are capable of digesting raw meat have jaws that go only vertical in motion. They can bite. Up and down. Herbivores grind their fiber meaning chewing not tearing and swallowing. Teeth in herbivores are flat to grind the fibers. Carnivores do not have flat teeth. For example, the dog does not have even one single flattened teeth. There are all sharp, and they are designed to tear the flash the same way the knife does. Also, no moving from left to right. Jaws muscles are stronger and much more pronounced. Humans have a small opening into the oral cavity and cannot swallow large chunks of meat. Trying to swallow large chunks, eating quickly, swallowing fibrous or poorly chewed foods often results in choking. Wolf for example, have a large opening to the oral cavity and can bite with most of the teeth at the same time and swallow larger chunks of meat. Normal bite force is around 400 pounds. In a situation where defending itself, a large wolf can bite down with a force that is equal to over 1,200 pounds of pressure. Rottie has a bite with 328 pounds of pressure, and the grown-up man can reach around 150 with the molars and 83 with incisors. The human incisors 83, wolf incisors 400. Human incisors are not for flesh. Their job is to tear or peel fiber and molars are for grounding. K9 teats and fangs are not for eating they are designed for killing. It is a weapon. Human K9's won't be able to kill. The K9 job is to go deep into the flesh and create internal bleeding by rupturing the arteries. There are weapons, and for example, gorilla K9's are at the same level as tiger ones. Tiger canine teeth also have very rich nerve endings. Tiger lore says that a tiger can sense the site of its prey's carotid arteries and target its bite to especially puncture them. Although strategies of predations can wary, predators will instinctively go for the neck because arteries there can be easily raptured. If a dog bites your leg probably he does not want to kill you or is unable to reach for the neck area. If you get attacked never go down. We can survive 30 bites to the arms and legs but one bite at the neck and game over.

Herbivore-style jaw joint is flexible and is designed for grinding vegetation, but it is a much weaker joint than the muscular carnivore one. The herbivore-style jaw joint would be easy to dislocate when attacking the prey. The fact that herbivore style joint is unable to withstand the stresses of subduing and struggling prey or to crush bones (nor would it allow the wide gape carnivores need) will, in reality, mean death. In the wilderness, an animal with a broken jaw would starve to death, therefore, be selected against. Also, the reality is that if species want to adopt weaker but more mobile herbivore-style joint, it has to be committed to an essentially plant-based diet. When we talk about omnivores like dogs, for example, we must understand that animal which catches prey need to have the physical equipment which makes predation practical and efficient. There can be no omnivore without that or at least true omnivore. Consequently, only real omnivore is the one of the carnivorous descent. Rest of us are just plant eaters that can stumble upon some termite or something similar.

Carnivore abdomen composition is more primitive than herbivorous adaptations. Therefore, one would expect an omnivore to be a carnivore that shows some adaptations of the gastrointestinal tract to an herbivorous diet. This is precisely the situation we found in the raccoons, the bears and some members of the canine families. Bears, for example, are mainly herbivores with 70-80% of their diet consisting from plant foods. Because bears include significant amounts of meat in their diet, they must maintain the anatomical characteristics that allow them to capture and kill their prey. Therefore, bears have a maxillary structure, musculature, and dentition that allow them to apply the forces necessary to kill and dismember their prey despite the fact that most of their diet consists of plant foods. The most important adaptation to an herbivorous diet in bears is the modification of their teeth. The bears kept the incisors, the large canines and the premolar shearers of a carnivore; but the molars were square with rounded cusps to crush and grind. They cannot digest the fibrous vegetation and, therefore, are highly selective. Their diet is dominated mainly by aromatic herbs, tubers, and berries. Many scientists believe that the reason why bears hibernate are due to their primary food (succulent vegetation) are not available in the cold winters of the north. The small intestine is short (less than five times the length of the body) like that of pure carnivores, and the colon is simple, soft and short. Moreover, when we look at the colon in general, the large intestine (colon) of carnivores and true omnivores is simple and very short, since its sole purpose is to absorb salt and water. It has almost the identical width as the small intestine and, consequently, has a limited capacity to function as a reserve. Although a microbial populace is still present in large amount in the colon of carnivores, its activities are essentially putrefactive.

In herbivorous animals, the large intestine is a highly specialized organ involved in the absorption of water and electrolytes, the production of vitamins and fermentation of plant fibers. The colons of herbivores are always more comprehensive than their small intestine and are relatively long and filled with probiotic bacteria. Microbiome of the colon in humans have an essential role in the normal functioning of the body. Somehow we underrate the importance of the colon and think it is just some waste material organ. In carnivores, it is, in us, it is not. In Homo sapiens and other primates colon is subject for a different array of functions. For example, water and electrolyte absorption and vitamin production and absorption. There is also extensive bacterial fermentation of fiber that results in the different metabolites and short-chain fatty acids production and absorption from the colon that also provides significant amounts of energy and other health benefits. We are not able to utilize the entire energy value of the fiber as grazers can do but we can utilize some of it. The extent to which the fermentation and absorption of metabolites take place in the human colon has only lately started to be studied, and research into microbiome is a new big thing because of all of the chemicals that these bacteria can secrete and effect that they have on our bodies. It is not just the vitamins that probiotic bacteria create. Every chemical is one possible drug. The composition of microbiome depends on the food we eat. One type ferment fiber another type purifies the meat, and not all of them are probiotic.

Think about it in this way, if bacteria putrefy the beans for example and we get gases as a result, it does not have a considerable interest in us. We are not her food. Bacteria likes the beans only. Bacteria are organisms that are specialized to a great extent. They do not eat everything as some individuals might think. One type eats fiber, other type eats meat. It likes you too but in a different way.

You are her host, and you give her all that food and place to live with moist and warmth so she may help you live longer because she likes you, but in a different way, she does not like your meat. However, when we have bacteria that putrefy corpses, then we are on the menu too. Meat is meat, and ours is tasty too. Most people do not realize that most of our immune system about 60-70% is actually in our abdomen as a vast system of lymph network referred to as GALT (gut associated lymphatic tissue).

Moreover, about 80% of plasma cells mainly immunoglobulin A (IgA)-bearing cells reside in GALT. We have more foreign DNA from bacteria and other symbiotic microorganisms in us than our own. In carnivores animals because of acidity most of the upper GI tract is sterile. When food reaches the colon, there can be no foreign invaders, and most of the already present species of colon microbiota are "nice" ones. When we eat meat situation is different. The human gastrointestinal tract features the anatomical modifications consistent with an herbivorous diet with low acidity and long transit time, so the potential for the growth of aggressive strains of not symbiotic bacteria is real, and if they are present in the food they can colonize the intestinal lining and cause constant presence for our immune system. The reason for the so-called balance between probiotic and non-probiotic bacteria is because of this. We always have a big chunk of our microbiome that is not symbiotic with our body. Eating meat feeds a large chunk of this nonsymbiotic bacteria. High animal products and low fiber consumption are not just associated with an increase of transit time and constipation. They are also associated with the rise of the low level of chronic inflammation and risk of colon cancer.

There is also a completely different mechanism that consumption of meat is associated with that will increase inflammation even if we do not count the live bacteria and all the toxins and drugs and pollution. This mechanism is natural and normal, and all of the carnivorous species had it, and the reason why this exists is because of the fact that even dead non-probiotic bacteria do count as toxins. These substances are known as endotoxins (Greek éndon within; cognate with Old Irish ind-), and the problem with them is that there are thermally (250C) and chemically stable and extremely toxic. Endotoxin is a complex lipopolysaccharide (LPS) found in the outer cell membrane of gram-negative bacteria (E.coli, Salmonella typhi, Shigella), typically waterborne. Bacteria shed endotoxin in large amounts upon cell death. Meaning, the bacteria can be dead or cooked for a long time, but their endotoxins are still there. Endotoxins are chemically very stable and can withstand both high temperatures and our bodies best attempts at acid and enzyme degradation. One of the leading causes of hundreds of studies that display enlarged inflammation from animal foods, but not from most plant foods, may be consequence of a toxic load of dead bacteria endotoxins in animal products. These bacteria secrete endotoxins that are absorbed into our system, leading to the endotoxemic inflammation we see after egg, meat and dairy consumption, as well. Fresh hamburger contains approximately a hundred million bacteria per quarter pounder. Eating meals high in bacterial endotoxins could develop mild but systemic inflammatory episodes that predispose subjects to the development of chronic diseases. The animal fat that comes in the same package may play a role in the pathogenesis of this after-meal inflammation. Endotoxins hold a powerful attraction for the saturated fat, so they stick to it and then get absorbed through the gut wall and into the bloodstream. Here is one study that discovered a link between endotoxin exposure and diabetes type 2 (High fat intake leads to acute postprandial exposure to circulating endotoxin in type 2 diabetic subjects doi: 10.2337/dc11-1593). This happens in animals too when they eat meat. What low level of inflammation does? It causes damage like any other inflammation just in prolonged period. What that translates to is faster and more noticeable DNA damage.

In contrast, plant foods do not show this trait, and actual consumption is correlated with the anti-inflammatory reaction after a meal because of the antioxidants and other anti-inflammatory phytochemicals. It would be interesting to see how much inflammation meat consumption causes in carnivorous species. So far I was unable to find research that looks into dead meat bacteria endotoxemia exposure in carnivorous species. This could be potentially interesting because if meat causes no inflammation in carnivorous animals, we might look at way how to lower the same inflammation in our own body.

There are still a number of differences that I want to mention. All creatures need to obtain their food in an energy efficient manner. Animals that are intended to eat plants are designed to forage. What that means is that their food is scattered over the large area, and they have to be able to cover vast areas in search for it and not just that, they are designed to eat for extended periods continually chewing on something. In order to do that moving must be cost efficient or energy expenditure will be higher than the calories that plant foods would provide and species will die. That is the reason why most of the herbivores including humans can stand and walk for hours with no problem. How can we stand for example in a job that requires it for 8 hours straight? There are species of herbivorous animals that can even sleep while standing. It is because our weight is held not by our muscles but with our bones. Our legs are straight. Weight distribution is held mostly by our skeletal structure and not by muscle tension. Muscles are there for moving and balance. Many people had argued why we adopted an upright stance. Energy cost of locomotion is to blame. For quadrupeds speed of locomotion and energy consumption is in direct linear codependence. The faster they move the more energy they consume. For humans, it is not. We consume less energy for locomotion then it would be expected for the animal of our size and gravity is to blame. For quadrupeds center of mass is always located in the center of the bases of support. That means every time a quadruped has to make a step he has to lift off his center of the mass and move it forward. When we want to make a step and lift our leg out our center of the mass is thrown outside of our body, and we start to fall forward.

Gravity is doing part of the work and helping us move. We are more efficient walker then apes and very efficient foragers.

As a consequence, the agility and speed are low. You can try to catch some small animal by hands and you will see what I mean. We are optimized for foraging. And of course, the meat eaters are optimized for predation. They do not have to cover large areas, but they do have a problem. What they hunt don't like to be eaten. What that means is running to catch the pray in short period. Why in a short period? Because predators must be quicker than the pray and they have to sacrifice something. That something is endurance.

They have something called digitigrade stance. Human and other primates ankles are even on the ground. Our knees are about in the midpoint of our legs. In digitigrade animals, it is only the toes that contact the ground while the ankle joint is well up off the ground. The knee is in fact in the upper 1/3rd of the leg. When predators stand up they are already in some sort ready to sprint mode because of their entire body weight stands on muscles. Their legs are bent in the joints. They have to use energy to resist gravity. They cannot stand or sprint or walk for extended periods. Even sitting requires muscle tension for dogs. For a dog to relax all of his muscles honestly, he must lay down. We have to walk our dog because of this, predators are at rest most of the time digesting meat, and when they have to hunt, they stand up and run. They are usually not successful. Average kill is about one in 7 to 10 days. Usually, the hunt is at night. They have at average 6 to 8 times better night vision than us. They have better all of the other senses too, except for color vision which is essential for identifying ripe and nutritious plant foods.

Herbivore, in contrast, is continuously standing and foraging. Because carnivore cannot run for extended periods like herbivores, they sneak up and seek weak, diseased, old, young or defective animals. This is predation mentality. In contrast, herbivores seek the opposite most colorful biggest and richest food because this food is most nutritious. Predation using herbivore mentality is destructive because it depletes the pray species gene pool of healthiest genes. This psychological difference was subconsciously embedded in our perceptions because it has to do with energy expenditure. Acquiring food takes much energy, and if that acquired energy is not significantly higher than the level that our body needs for functioning, acquired energy would not be able to sustain us, and we will be extinct. Efficiency is the essence of life. The more efficient we are, the more energy we have to spare for reproduction and other nice stuff in life. In inefficient hunting or foraging, the extinction is guaranteed. Carnivorous seek weakness to preserve energy at the same time herbivorous seek fullness to preserve energy by getting more energy balance from what they eat. Killing young, old, sick in any way weaker pray is also an evolutionary protective mechanism. On a picture, you can see two types of hunting, one real anatomically based hunting with real predator but also unnatural use of technology like an Aboriginal spear to catch the food that Aboriginal is not physiologically adapted to consume, especially in large amounts.

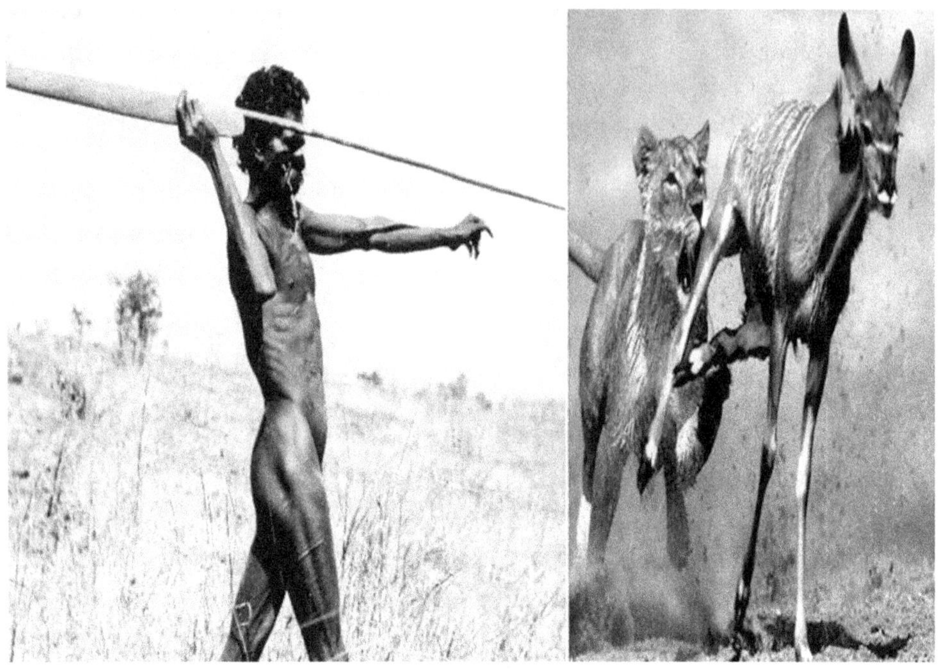

This is hard for people to grasp. I can try even to extrapolate this in sort of nasty Nazi theory. We as a species do not have natural predators anymore except our self to pray upon each other. That fact combined with modern human medicine spoils our gene pool. In the long run, because we now have hospitals and drugs to treat diseases and all of the technology, bad genes are no more selected against by nature. That would in time spoil our gene pool. If we understand this, let's call it predation theory, we will realize that we will become more and more sick with increases in all kinds of genetic disorders and infertility as time goes by.

Now because we have herbivore mentality what happens when we go out to hunt? We kill the biggest the best the healthiest animal we can find. Because we do not have a natural instinct for predation, we will kill everything we can get our hands on. We will deplete the world until there is nothing left. That is herbivorous mentality gone bad, and that is one of the psychological reasons why we do not care if we destroy our food supply because we are not the real predators no matter what some macho men think of himself. Real predators instinctively maintain their food supply. We destroy as any good grazer would graze until there is something to graze. When we look at some diseased chicken, we consider it to be ugly, bad and better to avoid. We like our chickens to be healthy with bright pink meat with no tumors and diseases inside. Real predator pursues exactly this sick, lame, ugly, old and stupid or just food that is already dead. Already dead and decomposing animal is just a free meal. No energy expenditure required. Some of them like wolves can smell diseased animals and single them out. This is the reason why dogs can be trained to sniff out cancer in patients. The energy content of the cancerous rotting corpse is exactly the same as nice pink in the middle one. When we see roadkill do we consider it to be an ideal situation for a little snack, or the smell of rotting corpse burns our eyes? Do our glands start to salivate in sight of blood? Most of us will agree that hunting if not necessary is activity no one will ever do if they have to risk injuring themselves. Only with modern weaponry, we have sports hunting that can be enjoyable experience. Level of cognitive development to advance technology is something Homo erectus did not have.

Furthermore, even if he did it would not make a difference in Africa without preservation techniques. Carnivores have one big single-chambered stomach. The volume of the stomach of a carnivore represents 60-70% of the total capacity of the digestive system. It is known that lions are capable of consuming as much as 90 pounds of meat in a single sitting. Since these animals only kill once a week on average, a large volume of the stomach is advantageous because it allows animals to quickly gorge as much as they can before other predators arrive. Also, they have to eat the entire kill to save the energy because if they only eat part of the kill, then they will have to hunt every day. They gorge themselves as much as they can at one time which can then be digested later while resting. Ninety pounds of meat is 60,000 calories. Human stomach holds about 25% of the capacity of the GI tract. In an adult, it is about 10 inches long and can quickly expand to hold as much as 1 quart (0.946 liters) of food with some estimates that it can go up to 2 liters of food. In comparison to a carnivore, it is tiny.

Carnivorous animals are designed for intermittent feeding while we are designed for constant feeding. If we count the energy content of natural foods human can consume about 900 to 1200 calories in a single sitting which is less than our caloric needs. What this means is that we must eat a couple of times during the day to our full stomach capacity or eat smaller portions throughout the day. Every single day. When carnivores eat, they consume enough energy to last them for a week, and this is important because they will probably not be successful in hunting every day. They can eat carrion no problem, the acidity of 1 is enough to dissolve not just bones but a metal penny too. When they kill they do not care about bacteria and viruses, and they will feed on the rotting corpse until they catch something else. For us and our hominin ancestors, small capacity of stomach and inability to eat carrion means we cannot retrieve a great amount of energy from the single carcass before it rots and a large amount of energy wasted for catching that pray will put us in deficit. Humans and Neanderthals even with the paleo technology would not be more efficient in hunting then carnivorous animals are. Even in modern times with all of the rifles, hunters are not successful every time they go hunting. Hunting will put us in energy deficit without preservation techniques. Only in icy climates hunting large animals will be energetically in surplus because the meat of the carcass will freeze before it goes bad. And that is the reason Neanderthals became omnivores in northern Europe from purely plant-eating lineage. In Africa, if we go around trying to catch something, and after ten days we are successful, we cannot even consume enough of calories at that one meal to replace all of the energy we spent before the meat goes bad. The only solution is fire. Before the roasting no meat for us. Even the cooked meat does not last for that long. Cooked meat or poultry at the Refrigerator (40 °F or below) has a storage time of 3 to 4 days. At insect infested hot Africa savannah, time for consumption before spoiling is much shorter and roasted leftovers are just baits for some large cat. If we do not catch something today and don't eat and then do not catch something in 10 days in the row, probably we will be too starving and exhausted to hunt again. The only way of hunting where metrics can work is in a larger type of the community of modern Humans or Neanderthals with labor division, but this requires high cognitive capability with advanced social structures and hierarchy with language, technology like fire, spears, clothing and so on.

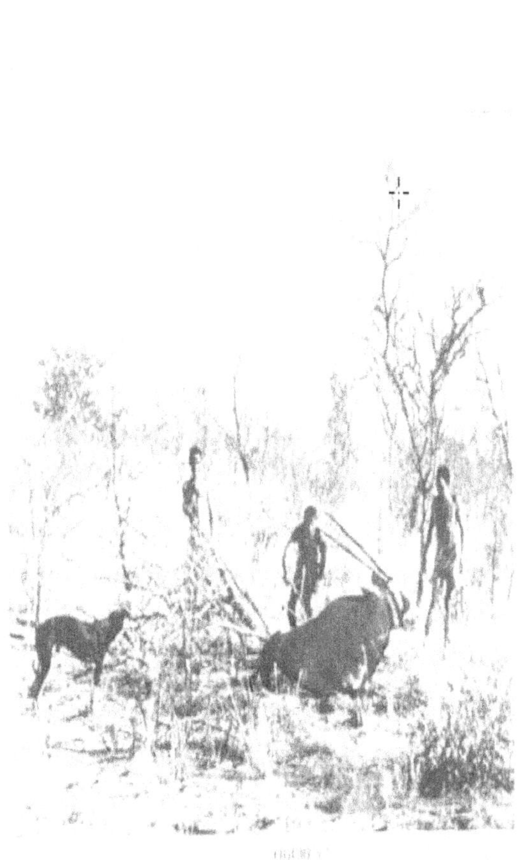

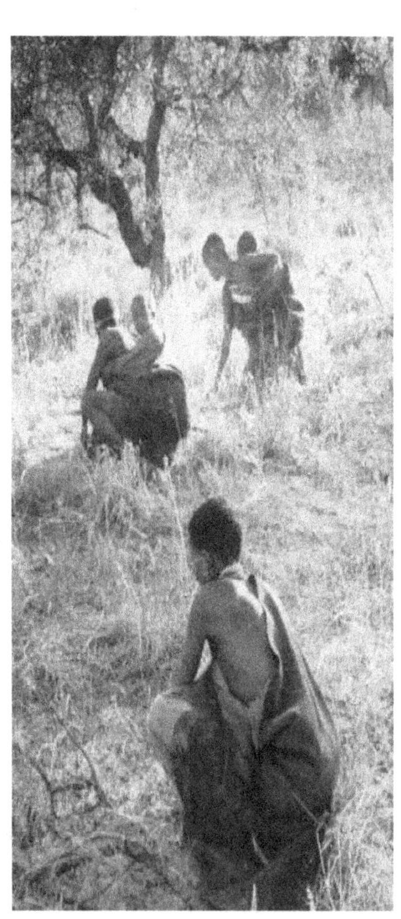

So how will metrics work? It goes something like this. A small group of hunters will go hunting. Not all of the men just small groups. Maybe one group or two depending on the size of the village. If the village is bigger more can go. They will go out to check the traps to see if anything smaller is trapped and then they will go hunting for something bigger like Antelope. Hunting can be directly killing or persistence hunting or something third. However, where the metrics work is that they will not eat the meat, they will bring it to the village for everyone to eat. Therefore, even if they themselves expended much of their energy and more than they can consume in the single sitting the entire village is in the surplus because that antelope will not last enough to get spoiled it will be eaten immediately by the entire village. In return when they are not successful hunters would eat regular food gathered from foraging by other tribe members.

This is a complex social structure. When we look at Africa tribes of today like Kalahari San people, for example, we can see something similar. Using poisons men can kill large and fast animals. Women have clever ways of rendering low-quality plant foods edible. Although archaeology suggests that the strategies used by San people is only a few thousand years old and is somewhat different from the strategies used by more ancient hunter-gatherers still it is on a similar line. When anthropologist looks at this, they will see a pattern that lasts 250,000 years to the time of Neolithic revolution and conclusion would be that this behavior is natural and that we are omnivorous as bears. And you will have thousands of books everywhere about paleo diet representing this short time period in human evolution as a basic human state. And the big question is how normal is this actually? Our physiology evolved from small plant-eating mammals for more than 60 million years, and we had been using this hunting strategy for 200,000 years. Does our body physiology really cope reasonably good with a larger quantity of meat? Russell Henry Chittenden, the father of American biochemistry, wrote back in 1904: "We hear on all sides widely divergent views regarding the needs of the body, as to the extent and character of food requirements, contradictory statements as to the relative merits of animal and vegetable foods; indeed, there is a significant lack of agreement regarding many of the fundamental questions that continuously arise in any consideration of the nutrition of the human body."

So what changed in 115 years? What is the conventional and natural diet for human beings? What is the food that enables us to look, feel, and function at our best? Not just to survive. Is it vegetarian or vegan? Does it contain meat? How much meat? To a large extent, we have the answers now just most of us do not want to hear it. Science is here, but unlike any other animal, we turned food into a drug for satisfaction. If we look at surviving, we can survive purely on raw meat if we cannot find anything else. However, that is not our optimal food. We had always turned to meat for survival, not for pleasure. That is a modern invention. If we analyze energy balance acquiring meat is a hazardous job if we do not have large scale animals to kill like mammoths. It is a situation of extreme necessity. I will give a real-life example of what this means.

I found that examples are something most people can relate. After World War 1, the civil war erupted in Russia led by communist rebellion. Russia had suffered six and a half years of World War I and then was engulfed in Civil War 1917–1922. In the book "What Is To Be Done?" one of the main points of

Lenin's writing was that a revolution can only be accomplished by the strong leadership of one or just a few select people at the top, over the masses and that workers must be controlled. He was not Marxist at full extent, the idea of eliminating social classes would not be possible in his view, and in his utopian society there would still be noticeable differences amid those in politics and the common worker. In another word, Bolsheviks did not care about people and wanted the power to rule over the masses. It was interesting that he was writing his book in capitalistic Germany with no issues. In deeply segregated Russian society after World War 1 civil war was the nail to the coffin. The droughts of 1920 and 1921 made the disaster even worse. The disease had reached epidemic proportions, with 3,000,000 people dying of typhus in the 1920s. The Russian economy and entire marketplace was destroyed by the war with destroyed factories and bridges, pillaged livestock and plundered raw materials with massive death rate from starvation, not "just" from massacres. In history this is known as the Russian famine of 1921-1922. The communists deliberately caused it because they believed that peasants were not on their side and were intentionally attempting to impair the war effort. A decision was made that the best way to deal with them is to starve them to death. The Bolshevik government had requisitioned supplies from the peasantry or stole them if you like with no compensation or in a minuscule amount in return. This has led farmers to reduce agricultural production drastically. Lenin ordered the seizure of food that farmers had cultivated for their livelihood and subsistence and their seed grain in retaliation for this "sabotage." This caused prompting widespread peasant revolts such as the Tambov rebellion of 1920-1921. It had numbers up to 70,000 and successfully defending the area against Bolshevik expeditions with numerous deserters from the Red Army that also joined the rebellion. It lasted until Bolshevik forces started to use a poisonous gas for liquidations of "bandits" and ended with seven concentration camps with mostly children, women and the elderly. Some of them were transferred to the encampments as hostages. Each month 15 to 20 percent of inmates in the camps died. So what would you do in the situation like this? Would you develop predation mentality? Millions of people have died. To survive, people had begun to seek weak, diseased, old and young. Everything that is weaker it can be a possible meal. And when I say animals, I count humans in there too. First animals to be eaten where regular cattle, pigs and chickens. Then cats and dogs. Then rats. Then when nothing was left humans came to the menu.

Because many had been dying from a disease, someone had an idea that because this is meat and if roasted it will be fine so when someone died from disease or was killed by some third party, cannibalism became the norm. Nothing was wasted. There were cases of corpses already buried being dug up. When this was not enough, people turned on their own families. They started eating their brothers, wives, children, parents. When this was not enough and eating already dead family members could not sustain them any longer, killing started. And not just by moms and dads killing their children and eating them but also children themselves were killing their younger siblings for food. And there is still to come. There is something even worse than this, and I doubt that you can figure out what can be worse than 10-year-old boy killing his 3-year-old sister and eating her flesh. This practice had become so widespread that it became normal. No police no nothing. Just the new meat markets.

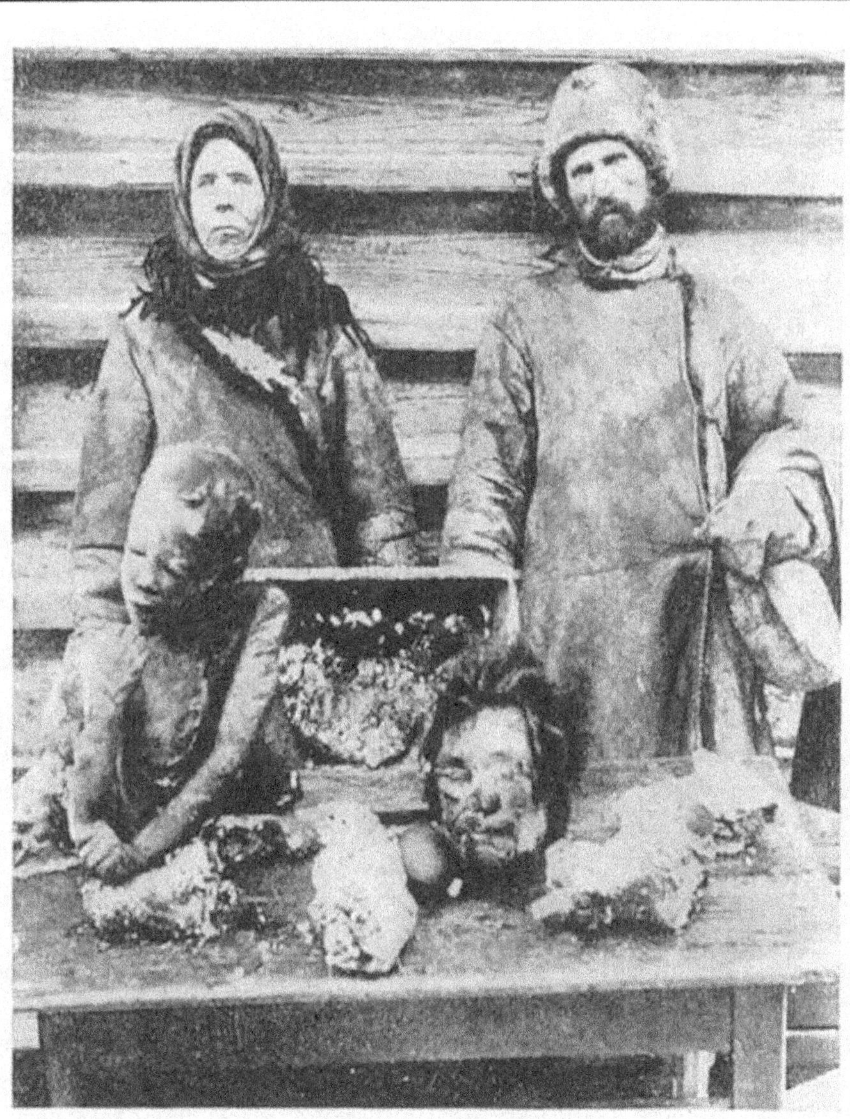

Стоит слева — Акулина Чугунова: зарезала живьем 6-летнюю дочь и половину ее съела. Стоит справа — Андрей Семыкин: разрубил на части умершую от тифа квартирантку и съел ее. Впереди — остатки съеденных ими трупов

Translation from Russian: "On the left Akulina Chugunova slaughtered her six-year-old daughter and ate half of her. On the right Andrei Semykin cut up into pieces a lodger who died from typhoid and ate him, in front are remains of corpses that they ate." Because practice became normal and of course if you have some more meat you can sell it. You can sell your half-eaten daughter and some severed heads; there is no problem. In starvation, meat is meat and nothing is wasted, and like any other predators in extreme conditions, people start looking at sick, lame, ugly, old and stupid or just food that is already dead. This is predation mentality. If we are healthy and full of life, we are not food anymore we are a danger to be avoided. Why? Because we are already ourselves on the brink of death, and sick, and if we get in trouble with someone who is stronger than us we can end up on the plate in his home.

That is why it is most "reasonable" to eat our children first and dig up some corpses before we try to kill someone else, or if we found some carrion, well good for us. Hollywood has all of this walking dead apocalypse movies where we get good adrenalin rush watching it eating popcorn. Maybe we should look at the mirror. Meat is not our number one food choice, and it is a form of extreme diet and always has been the diet for extreme conditions for survival. It was always expensive and just 100 years ago most of the masses, if we count out the royalty, could afford it only on holidays like Christmas and Thanksgiving. Rest of the year it was just regular vegan food, rice, potatoes, corn, and bread. The same situation exists even today in most of the third world countries where poverty is prevalent. Rural China, India, Africa. Most of the people still are surviving on cheap starch food. Only in developed countries, the situation is different. Eating meat is considered a healthy trait because poor people cannot afford it so individuals that are successful can eat it every day and if possible three times a day.

In China, for example, we have a situation that brown rice is not suitable anymore. In the past Chinese emperors had only eaten nice white rice and peasants has sustained themselves on brown. When peasants today come to new factories in big new cities to work they do not like to eat brown anymore. They can afford white, and although brown is healthier, they still don't want to eat it. It is peasant food. This psychology of social acceptance is what drives anxiety of carnism. If you feel that you are not fully satisfied if you do not eat animal protein in a meal you might have an anxiety disorder. In extreme cases, it can blow up to become an extreme form of diet that thrive primarily on animal protein. The "reason" is that animal protein is good for you. The highest of all quality of all food that exists on this planet, the chicken breast, salmon and low-fat beef that only successful people can afford. Eating starch is for losers. In a country where I live is exactly like this. Low meat consumption is correlated with famine and disease and poverty. When I started to lower my animal products consumption I was getting negative at some cases even hateful reactions with comments like: "Your teeth are going to fall out." "You are in the sect you need to seek some professional help." At that time and most of my life, I was eating mostly dairy products and meat for every meal in different forms with some veggies here and there.

I do not tell people what I eat in my personal life. I am not kidding. I do not tell people what my diet is. I do not care about wasting energy. This book is for individuals that already want to know and seek the knowledge and answers. It is not for "masses," and I do not care. You should live in every way that you like. I am not an advocate. My book is for people who have the desire to learn. Also, don't use material from book to convince family or friends or anyone into anything. If there is already desire for learning, then you can. To understand fully why is most "reasonable" to eat our children first we can look into experiments that researched psychological reaction to hunger. The psychological reaction to hunger is also what makes dieting useless in the long run and what subconsciously shapes our perception.

One of the first scientific studies on what hunger does to the mind was observed in a study remembered as the Minnesota Starvation Experiment performed by the University of Minnesota back in 1944. The lead investigator was Ancel Keys who had two Ph.D.'s one from biology and one from psychology. Thirty-six men were selected that were healthy and had no eating disorders from hundreds that volunteered. It was a study where the goal was to live on the diet of 1500 calories for six months. In the first 12 weeks there was 3200 calories control period, and then a real experiment started. Now 1500 calories are far from real starvation. American government wanted to understand what psychological and physiological effects are going to be on war-torn Europe with starvation and holocaust. Men were housed in a basement in the Minnesota University stadium in windowless rooms with a program of mental and physical exercises. Diet was strictly controlled, and they could not cheat because they were in some sense incarcerated for six months. They started to lose weight and by the end of the study they lost a significant number of pounds, but also it had psychological effects on them. In the beginning, they started to be apathetic, irritated and they developed ritualized eating patterns. Putting water into potatoes in order to make them bigger. Holding the food in the mouth and chewing for an extended period. Licking the plates. Daydreams of food, chewing gum, smoking cigarettes until someone had 30 packs per day. Drinking a ton of water to fill their stomachs. Then they started to enjoy solitary activities and looked at food in sexual manner. They had no regular sex drive and was only interested in what people ate. They developed an eating disorder mentality. Started to feel bad about themselves if they binge and felt guilt with food. What they considered normal weight before, during the study was considered to be overweight. When they look at their old pictures, they thought they have big stomachs and much more weight than what will in that situation for them be normal human physique. They experienced confusion when they are hungry and also when they are not. This is an extract from one off the volunteer's diary: "I am beginning to isolate myself from the other subjects. We are developing all kinds of weird behaviors. Everyone seems to be losing their interpersonal skills and starvation is less than half over. One of them bit the other volunteers. Many tried to escape from the compound to eat grass from nearby gardens. Another became so deranged that he chopped three of his fingers off with an ax." Later the ax men stated that he was messed up and that he could not remember why or how he chopped his fingers, and he could not say that he did not do it on purpose. This is what strict diet of 1500 calories did to this person in less than six months. What happened after the experiment is even more important.

When they started to feed on their own wish, Key noticed something entirely unexpected. They rapidly put on weight but not only that. They gained more than what they had on the starting point. Dieting made them fatter. They experienced something called extreme hunger. They ate and ate and ate and ate and never felt satisfied. Most companies in the diet industry and medical care know about this. Dieting can make you fatter. Fear of starvation is real. Fear of not having animal protein is real. Psychophysical dependence on supernormal stimuli is real. Human beings are evolutionarily conditioned for extreme eating because of the scarcity in nature. We have been consuming meat as part of our diet for 250,000 years, and likely we will not change this behavior until the last living animal is gone from the earth. To make things worse, at the same time, Humankind does not show the anatomical characteristics that one expects to find in anatomical omnivores such as raccoons and bears. Consequently, we have to pay the price for our choices. Usually, it comes with the medical bill.

Carnism is a word that Melanie Joy, Ph.D. used to define the value system and norms that define the dominant meat-eating culture. Meat eating is the culture that is learned. Actual carnivore would eat any meat no matter what it is. In our system, we would eat only a few animals that we deem as food. For example, would you eat your dog? The average intelligence of the pig is at the level of the 3-year-old child, and the pig is more intelligent than a dog. Pig is a very smart animal. Do we think that dog meat does not have a good taste? In China, they do eat dogs. Golden Retriever stew. Sounds delicious.

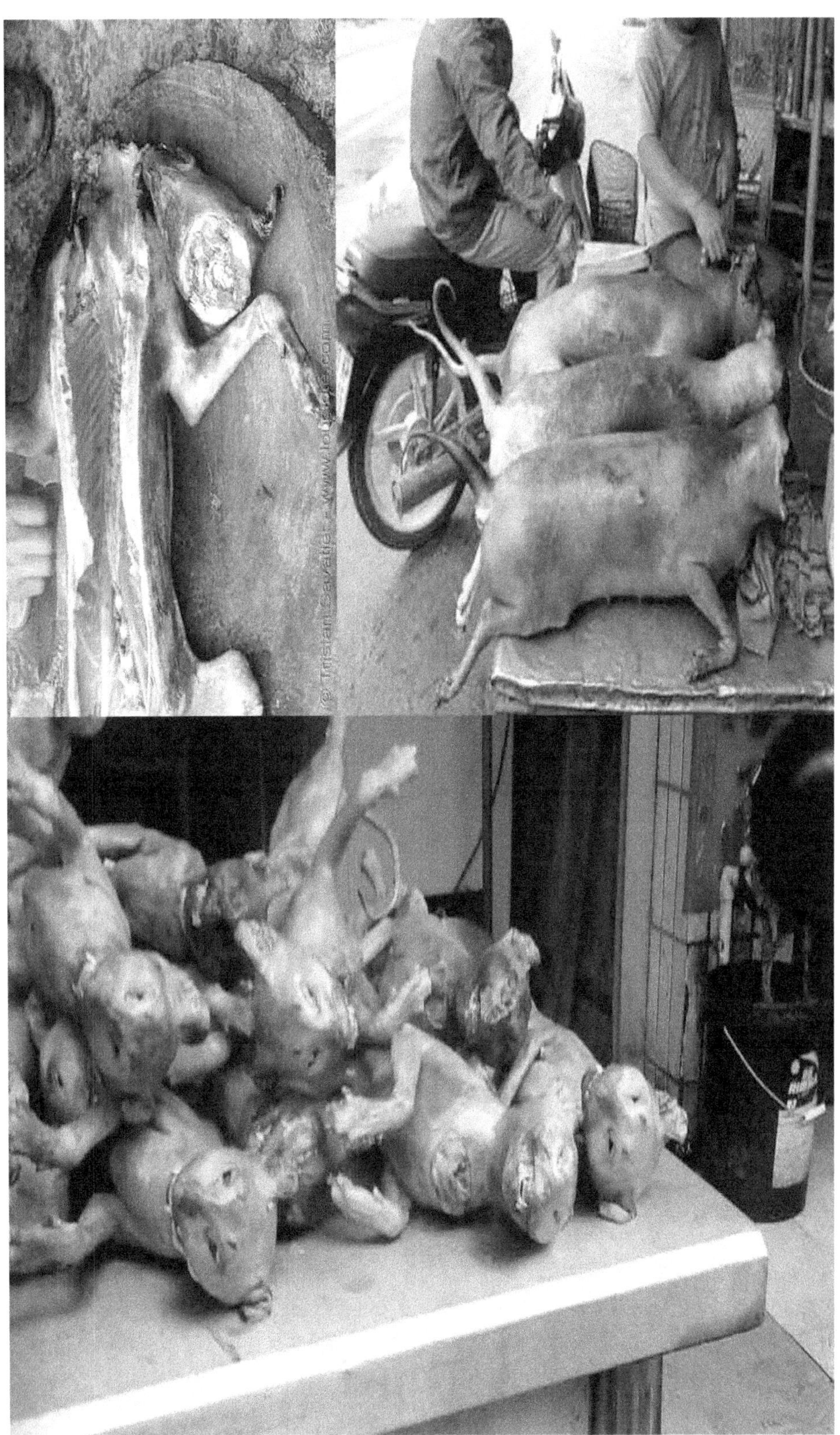

So why don't we eat them? Why not human meat? Do we think that human meat does not have good taste? In the words of Alexander Pearce, an Irish convict notorious for cannibalizing his fellow prison escapees: "Man's flesh is delicious, it tastes far better than fish or pork." Alternatively, how about this: "It was like good, fully developed veal, not young, but not yet beef. It was very definitely like that, and it was not like any other meat I had ever tasted... It was mild, good meat with no other sharply defined or highly characteristic taste such as for instance, goat, high game, and pork have."- William Seabrook, an explorer who ate a human rump steak on a trip to West Africa. In more recent times science presenter Greg Foot was trying to get to the secret of what human flesh tastes like in an experiment with BritLab for the BBC. Unfortunately, it is illegal to eat our own flesh. Having understanding that it is illegal the entire end goal was to experience some resemblance of the taste. They performed a biopsy of Greg's leg muscle and settled for the aroma of his cooked flesh. Aroma of the flesh can account for up to 80 percent of our sensation of taste. They put the cooked human meat in aroma analyzing machine and did the smell test. In Greg words, his leg muscle smelled like beef stew. Analysis of the leg muscle showed that it is very similar in composition to both chicken and beef. It is about half of the muscle we found in chicken breast and have similar muscle fiber we found in cuts of beef. In the end, they created a ground meat mixture of different animal meets to recreate the fibers they found in the biopsy of his leg and made a fake human burger. Cannibalism is thoroughly documented around the world, from Amazon Basin to the Congo, Fiji and the Maori people of New Zealand. It is not a modern invention, and in some cultures, it is normal. There is ceremonial ritual cannibalism also. In the modern world it was still practiced in Papua New Guinea as of 2018 in ceremonial rituals and the war ceremonies in various Melanesian tribes. Neanderthals are believed to have practiced cannibalism. Anatomically modern humans may have also eaten Neanderthals.

On the smaller farms, slaughter is always done with bare hands without anesthesia. Same with any other animal. Male chicks do not lay eggs and don't grow quickly enough so after hatching they are selected and put into grinding machine while still alive. Females are sent to a hot blade to remove part of the chicks beaks. After debeaking, birds are put into cages where they are going to spend the rest of their lives confined in tiny space. Because of selective breeding, they are grown to be so large so quickly that many suffer crippling leg disorders and chronic joint pain. At the slaughter plant birds are snapped upside down into moving shackles by their legs and then pulled across a blade witch slices their throats.

Humane meat is a just humane myth. No matter if we are talking about chickens or pigs or any other animal. It is like saying humane concentration camp. And at the end, they are just stupid pigs wright. Well wrong. Pigs are at least as intelligent as a three-year-old human child, cows develop deep and lasting bonds with their family and friends, chickens are able to distinguish more than

100 different faces of the members of their species and have 30 different calls to signal different frets. Animal cognition is a vast topic.

From Kanzi the bonobo to Akeakamai the dolphin it would take an entire chapter to begin to analyze it. Kenzi, for example, learned more than 500 lexigrams. Even more importantly he was able to connect these lexigrams to represent a form of small sentences. In a study done back in 1993, he performed better than a human 2-year-old at responding to verbal requests. Akeakamai and Phoenix, his tank mate dolphin, were taught how to recognize words. Akeakamai was taught words that were represented by different gestures made by the hands of a human trainer. Phoenix learned by listening to words through computer-generated electronic sounds. These sounds were reproduced through an underwater speaker. Both dolphins have successfully learned individual words and eventually strings of words or sentences. Impressively, the dolphins could understand the instructions given with different grammatical structures and different word orders. They understood the difference between instructions like "Take the hoop to the ball" and "Take the ball to the hoop." When they performed the required actions correctly, the dolphins showed that they understood the elements of the language. This is intelligence at the level of humans. Even more remarkably, the dolphins seemed to be able to collaborate creatively. Human managers asked the dolphins to come up with their own trick together, using the tandem and create commands. The dolphins responded with a synchronized behavior of their choice, such as diving backward or squirming their tails. Militaries of the world even trained and experimented with dolphins with the idea to create soldiers out of them. Dolphins are at the level of cognition vary closely matching to humans. However, this fact is irrelevant to us.

Cognition has nothing to do with it. In Japan, they like to eat dolphin meat. They like to kill them just because they are competition. It is all about exterminating as much of them as possible in order to make the oceans fish available to fisherman. A form of pest control. We in the western world like to watch the tricks they learned in their prison tank at the amusement park. When we say a stupid pig or retarded chicken, it is just a form of justification. It is just that we consider in our culture pig meat as a food source and dog meat as not. We will dress and love our dogs and eat our pigs. The truth is that most animals can think and feel and do have a high level of cognition or at least higher than we would like them to have. It is a well-documented observation that domestic animals, especially dogs in some cases refuse to vacate locations where they last saw their masters. In nature, there are recorded cases of wild animals that revisit their dead and linger over them. There are many cases of wild animals that adopt orphans of same and also other species. For example, elephants have a wide range of what we might consider human emotions like grief and post-traumatic stress. They can cry from grief too. Same as chimpanzees and humans, they grieve and bury their dead. They are also exhibiting a great deal of interest for the bones of their own kind. In some occasions, elephants that are entirely unrelated to the departed still visit their graves. They are frequently seen gently investigating the bones while remaining very quiet. Elephant researcher Martin Meredith had described in his book the usual elephant death ritual. "The entire family of a dead matriarch, including her young calf, were all gently touching her body with their trunks, trying to lift her. The elephant herd was all rumbling loudly. The calf was observed to be weeping and made sounds that sounded like a scream, but then the entire herd fell incredibly silent. They then began to throw leaves and dirt over the body and broke off tree branches to cover her. They spent the next two days quietly standing over her body. They sometimes had to leave to get water or food, but they would always return." This type of elephant behavior around humans is also typical in Africa. It is well documented that they have buried dead humans too or that they had aided them when they were hurt. Because of this type of behavior elephants are thought to be highly altruistic animals. In India, in one case an elephant was working with the locals in a construction site. He was lifting the logs from the truck and then placing them in pre-dug holes. At the particular hole, he suddenly refused to lower the log. When the mahout (elephant trainer) came to investigate the hold-up, he noticed that a dog was sleeping in the hole. Only after the dog got out to the safety, the elephant lowered the log. Scientists often debate the extent to which elephants feel the emotions and any other animal for that manner. If species refuses the order of his master to save the life of another species in my mind at least, this is a representation of intelligence and awareness.

A few years ago an elephant caw named Zhuang Zhuang made headlines and broke hearts when a video of him made it online. Baby elephant cried for 5 hours after being rejected and stamped on and repeatedly kicked and almost killed by its mother. However, the real question here is: Was Zhuang Zhuang cried emotional tears? At the point when rhesus monkeys are separated from their mothers, one of their most common reactions is to cry. When dogs are lost or isolated from their caretakers, they too can shed tears. For a long time scientist thought that animals do cry emotional tears, but the evidence was anecdotal. Charles Darwin even wrote a book on the topic in which he had an entire chapter about weeping Asian elephant that he was convinced was showing human-like emotion. Today situation is different. Most of the animal behaviorists think that animal crying might be a hired wired response to lack of contact or stress and not an emotional reaction. In my mind, a lack of social contact is an emotional reaction like when you get lost as a child and start to cry, but in their mind, it is not. It is hired wired response to stress.

By performing brain scans on animals like monkeys, dogs, and rodents, a group of animal behaviorist can compare brain activity with the activity of the human mind. There are trying to figure out does animal brains look like human brains when human brains feel certain emotions. So far results show that animal brainwaves do look a lot like human brainwaves when we are experiencing fear, anger or joy. They even reacted in a comparable fashion to displays of emotion in others. It is a form of empathy that numerous specialists previously thought to be unique only to modern humans. In one research from primate researchers in Japan, (Brain response to affective pictures in the chimpanzee. doi:10.1038/srep01342) investigators estimated event-related brain potentials (ERPs) in conscious chimps as they watched at images of either emotional or neutral faces. The results revealed a differential brain potential is appearing 210ms after the introduction of a compelling image. It is the same pattern we can see in modern humans. This implies that at least a limited part of the emotional system is similar both in chimpanzees and humans. This result if we disregard all religious and social factors hold implications for the evolutionary foundations of emotional phenomena, such as emotional cognition and empathy. The chimpanzees, as it turns out, show the brain pattern identical to that of their human counterparts when they look at emotional images. Even if they cannot vocalize at the same level that we can what they are thinking, the underlying emotional process might be similar to what we term universal human emotion. Why would we presume any differences in brain patterns in elephants or dogs? The truth is that we do not really care or ever would. Animals may have empathy, but humans have selective empathy. We may feel bad for dogs but not for pigs, and we may feel bad for dead children casualties of war but not when it is our bombs that did the damage. Then it is called collateral damage, and we do not think about it. It is something I like to call selective comprehension.

Dr. Melanie Joy calls it a gap in our consciousness, the block of awareness. A form of denial or self-defense mechanism. She talks about three ends of justification. The eating meat is healthy, normal and necessary. However, what we think is normal is the just social structure of the dominant culture. For most of the time of the entire human existence slavery was normal, natural and necessary. Even in the Christian Middle Age Europe with the inquisition, slavery was normal and natural. Slave trade was even necessary for the economy of the newly ethnically cleansed territories of the new world. In one hand we hold a holy bible and talk about puritanism. In another hand, we have guns to kill native Americans and ships to bring us black Africans to work on our plantations. There are just "savages" that run naked. Well for most of human history running naked was running natural. Clothing is a modern invention. And what is natural represent the dominant culture interpretation of history? Murder, rape, infanticide, abortion, and child sacrifice were all natural for most of the human history. And what is slavery? Serfs in the Middle Ages during serfdom were required to work for the lord of the manor who owned that land. In return, they had the right to protection, justice and the right to cultivate specific fields for their own sustenance. Serfs were often asked not only to work in the lord's fields but also in forests, mines and to work to maintain roads. Workers of today are not required to work for the lord or anything else. However, there are required not to steal and have to pay with money to maintain their substance. What happens when money supply runs out? In all practical meaning most of the population, today works for the lord's owned companies and banks and have mortgages student loans and debts. The only difference is that serfs were usually working between 6 am, and 12 am and then own the remainder of the day to be free, and for entire winter there is no working on the fields. So they have a big winter holiday. Workers of today work 8 hours a day plus transportation and have 15 days a holiday two times a year. Serfs had much more free time. If we think we are free, try to go to nature and live off the grid. Even if you physically are capable and know what you are doing it is illegal to do so.

Human is the only animal who is bound to pay with money for its existence and not allowed to live in his natural state in the wilderness. If you try to do that, then the system will not like it and would send its armed members to catch you and to put you in a cage. If you are not part of the system, then you are a danger to the system. You are not free to live self-sufficient life outside of the grid. It is illegal in most of the countries in the world. It is illegal if you do not have an id card. First id card in the history was introduced and forced on the population by Nazi Germany in order to have the ability for identification of Jews on the street. "By establishing a peoples registration (Volkskartei – ID card) we will achieve complete supervision of the entire German people" -Herman Göring, 1938, quoted in The Nazi Census. In common law countries so far everywhere we look in the entire world no common law country has accepted an obligatory peacetime identification system. However, the situation is changing. Now we have biometric id cards and cameras everywhere and satellites that can zoom in to take a picture of our face. Every transaction with a credit card is saved, every email we sent is saved, everything is tracked. There is no running away. Dominating other animals to our will and not caring about it is no different from dominating another human animal to our will and don't care about it. There is one good quote from Mahatma Gandhi: "The greatness of a nation can be judged by the way its animals are treated." This can be truthful because patterns of behaviors are usually the same and do not change. Only selective awareness changes for justification of behavior. The mentality of violence and domination is the same. They even put Dr. Michael Greger's Nutritionfacts.org website on the list of sites created and funded by the Russian government to undermine US elections. There is a website called proper not created by intelligence community who does "meticulous" research to identify "tools" of Russian propaganda. I was laughing when I saw that but not for very long. The intelligence community does not make mistakes. They later removed it from the list. It is a large community with lots of regular people who do not understand the system that started to ask the questions like why and how. The reason is that they just don't like someone messing with their industries. Many people who tend to think tent to go toward science-based nutrition and then ask more than they should so they, or me, or you are a potential terrorist. Again everything that is not in line with the system is against it. Actually, all you read here is just Russian propaganda.

Also, just in case if you may have some idea of rescuing some piglets, today it is not just breaking and entry and stealing. In 2008 the FBI wrote: "Together, eco-terrorists and animal rights extremists are one of the most serious domestic terrorism threats in the U.S. today." The U.S. is so concerned with animal rights extremism that there is specific legislation for them: The Animal Enterprise Terrorism Act (AETA). No other terrorist act targets a specific ideology. The law was created in 2006 with intent to expand the governmental power to enable the investigations to have legal right to look for all unwanted terrorist activities meaning they will arrest people based on their speeches and internet posts. In 2006, a man was sentenced to three years for conspiracy to commit crimes under AETA based on speeches he gave, forum posts and participation in protests. Just so that we can understand, free speech and liberty are not when we get arrested for internet forum posts and speeches no matter what they are. It is something called thought crime. Like in the George Orwell novel 1984. Many of the people of the vegan community believe that treatment of animals is a social justice issue. That is exactly what for example Dr. Melanie Joy teaches on her lectures. If she is not high-level profile same as Dr. Gregor, she will get herself charged with domestic terrorism charges in no time. The more we will learn the more we understand the nature of human existence. And there is nothing evil about it. Subjugating others weaker to our will is the essence of existentialism. It is the driving force that drove most of human society in the ancient world, the classical world, the medieval world, and colonial exploitation. Existentialism is the force that drives all animals and evolution. Self-preservation, self-interest no matter what. Psychopathy at its best.

What most of the emotional people from vegan communities do not understand is that selective awareness is not just a defense mechanism. It is evolutionary instinctive subconscious self-preservation instinct. The only reason, for example, we do not eat dogs is not because we somehow culturally learned not to, but because we had more use of them alive. It is self-interest again. We have used dogs for hunting to catch other animals, and we used them as some form of primitive alarm system. They will bark when bear or wolf or other human or Neanderthal cross into our territory because wolfs are territorial animals and dog, is part of the human pack now. The tendency we have to not eat cats is not that we learned it culturally. It is because they are a form of primitive pest control. Cats tend to eat rats, so we had more benefit from domesticating them instead of eating them. In time behavior merges with our culture and became integrated into social norms. The same reason we do not like pigs is that they do not bark, they do not catch rats, they don't do anything. We have no benefits from them, they are "stupid", and we are going to eat them. If we try to milk them, that will not be good also because they are relatively small. Cattle, in contrast, are larger so no pig milk for us. The only reason we even have civilization is that primitive hominids like Homo erectus had more benefits from cooperating than living like a lone wolfs on their own. Hominins to had villagers or communities because it benefited the individual. Even a beta male will tolerate the alpha male not because it feels good to be beaten but because it is more beneficial for him to be beta then to go lone wolf. Everything ever conducted by any animal including humans come down to preservation instinct and existentialism. And then it became part of cultural norms. Telling people not to eat animals because it is murder, I am sorry to say this but grow up. Society structure is based on murder and force and hierarchy.

Exact nature of existence for any animal comes down to two things. Evasion of pain and death is the primary force. When that is taken care of then seeking of pleasure becomes the purpose. That is it. People are going to eat other people and animals and anything they can get their hands on if it is necessary or feels pleasurable. Also, meat and food, in general, is a form of the drug. It may be problematic to explain to your daughter that that chunk of meat she likes is, in fact, part of little Bambi that hunters killed but she needs to grow up sometime. Carnism is so entrenched in the psyche that fear of not having animal protein in every single meal can become a form of the anxiety disorder. The brief part of human evolution in-between hominin ancestry and Neolithic revolution made an impact. For a big chunk of our modern time around 250,000 years, we did eat meat in statistically important quantities. However, from the Neolithic revolution, we did not. A number of people start to rise so any foraging would not be sustainable. We have the same situation now. Without agriculture, with just hunting wild beast and fishing there would be widespread famine. In some areas of the world, the population reached peaks where even one dry season can create supply problems, and import of food products is the must. The same thing happened after the Neolithic revolution.

Dr. McDougall had one good remark explaining his starch-based diet that all prosperous civilizations on the world in history that existed and became known were based on starch. Whether it is corn and yucca among Native Americans, potatoes in South America, millet in Africa, barely in the Middle East, rice in Asia, or sorghum in East Africa, human civilization has been powered by starch throughout history. This is absolutely true. Starch-based diet is not the best one, but it is not the worst one either. If I had to rank it, I would say that it is better than 80 percent of other diets. Not ideal but reasonably ok. It can sustain a human organism without causing significant diseases. When I say or he says starch, that does not mean white flour or cornstarch. It means whole food items that have based its energy uptake on storing complex carbohydrates in them. Seeds store energy as fat, grains as starch, fruit as sugar. Also not all starch is the same.

Grains are easily digestible by humans even in the raw form because of saliva enzymes. First, our sense of smell is going to let our brain know that we are about to eat. This signal the glands in our mouth to secrete saliva. An enzyme called amylase is responsible for the breakdown of starch. Starch consist of amylose 20% and amylopectin 80%. As a primary enzyme in saliva, it begins the process of digestion by breaking down starches into the maltose from amylose and dextrin from amylopectin. Starches are long chains of simple sugars attached to each other, and amylase breaks the bonds along the chain to release maltose and dextrin molecules. If you want to experiment, you can chew on a cracker for a couple of minutes, and you will find that it will start to taste sweet. Some food can be eaten raw like grains but others cannot.

If we want to eat beans, for instance, this process is not posable if beans are not cooked, and they cannot be digested. Sprouted beans can be eaten by the way. For all the preppers out there, beans have enzymes that kill the putrefying microorganisms so they will not rot for an extended period if kept in dry storage. They can be sprouted and eaten after a day in row form. If you want to cook beans sprout them to deactivate all the bad enzymes first. However, still beans are not 100 percent digestible, and they will partially go unabsorbed all the way to our colon causing fermentation. We are more designed for grains and seeds then for beans but if we can tolerate flatulence beans are very healthy too. Even today when we realistically look on the food items that are consumed, most of the human population is relying on starch. The more undeveloped the nation, the more starch predominated diet. Because of this in the minds of some individuals, starch must be unhealthy poor people starvation food. The reason is terrible logic. I said in the first chapter that percentage is the key. It is the percentage of calories of animal products we eat. It is a percentage of time in our evolution that we had been eating them plus the relative percentage of calories we had been able to get from them in the overall diet in our evolution. There are still parts of the world where poverty is typical, and people still live in the line of their ancestors where industrialization have not yet taken place like rural China and India and Africa. There are studies done that looked into the correlation between this form of diet and so-called western diet. We can check to see what diseases these people have by eating nothing but rice or nothing but potatoes. Moreover, we can trace the diet change and health rate change when the standard of living goes up, for example, like in Okinawa. Some of the people who were poor also ended up migrating to developing countries, and we can see shifts in their health status as soon as they adopt a western diet with animal protein.

Maybe one of the most extensive studies in this field was The China–Cornell–Oxford Project. A large observational study conducted in rural China in the 1980s, co-financed by Oxford University, Cornell University and the Government of China. The study was comprehensive and included 367 different variables. A total of 65 counties in China with 6,500 adults were examined with a medical examination, blood tests, questionnaires, etc. In 1983 two random villages were chosen in each of the 65 rural counties of China and 50 families were randomly selected in each village. The eating habits of one adult member of each family, half men and half women were examined. The results were compared with mortality rates in those counties for 48 forms of cancers and other diseases during 1973-75. It was one of the most significant studies ever done known as The China Study. I will use some quotes from the study. "When we were done, we had more than 8,000 statistically significant associations between lifestyle, diet, and disease variables." "The results of these, and many other studies showed nutrition to be far more important in controlling cancer promotion than the dose of the initiating carcinogen." And not just breast cancer that was almost none existent but many other forms of cancers also. They even had a difficult time finding women who know other people who had breast cancer. People who were living in this rural areas of China known about the disease but have never seen it. No acne for example either. Many diseases and cancers are associated with hormones like IGF-1. I will write more about it in the chapter about protein in part two of the series. No diabetes too and I am not kidding. They were eating nothing but rice and still, diabetes was no concern. Paleo diet people have a hard time with that one. They believe the white rice is correlated with diabetes like any other refined carbohydrate. Then no heart disease, and so on. "People who ate the most animal-based foods got the most chronic disease. People who ate the most plant-based foods were the healthiest." Whether you become vegan or not, they suggest you put as many plants as possible on your plate at every meal. The study concluded that the counties with high consumption of food of animal origin in 1983-84 were also expected to have higher mortality rates from western diseases, while the opposite was true for the counties that consumed more plant-based food.

Now we can say this is maybe not related to their diet because there is a lot of other factors like exercise. These people mostly do manual labor, and maybe that was what sustained them. There were other variables too. Also, again this is not the only study of this kind. The problem with this kind of data is that goes against the interests of the industry, and because it is a significant study, it can be a hard time disproving it. What they do is usually make false logic knowing that most of the people do not really care and need to hear something they like to justify themselves their unhealthy behaviors. There is a good quote from T. Colin Campbell in The China Study that said: "Americans love to hear good things about their bad habits." For example, after the book, The China Study was published and made an impact, the written debate came. In 2008, "nutritionist" Loren Cordain argued that: "The fundamental logic underlying Campbell's hypothesis (that low [animal] protein diets improve human health) is untenable and inconsistent with the evolution of our own species." She argued that there are cultures like Maasai people and the Eskimos that do not suffer from health issues described by the authors which are entirely false by the way. So the study is false. However, wait. How far does the evolution of our species go? It is highly unlikely that educated people like her do not understand how evolution works. Maybe evolution goes as much as we need it to go so that we can justify our agenda. This is an inversion in the purest form. Nothing to do with science. This kind of behavior is a form of indirect murder, and we find this all over the modern medical industries. They are not there to heal you there are there to lie to you so you would be confused and then chronically ill and be a good customer. Walking zombie. Just stop lying to yourself, you have dealings with lying doctors all the time. They make a living by prescribing medicine. They are just salesmens for big pharma. People like nutritionist Loren Cordain know very well what real evolution look like they are not idiots. You are. In part 2 of the book series, you would read how much corruption exists in the field of medicine. For every single one study, we will have doctors with Ph.D.`s popping up like mushrooms with their authority and white coats trying to mud the water with different data just enough to make confusion knowing well enough that people do what feels good not what is right. There were charges against Campbell that he distorted and misrepresented the data from the study and that he had numerous flaws in his reasoning. The problem was it was just statistical correlations. His work is actually not that of a big deal. There were other similar statistical studies and studies in biochemistry that later proved most of this statistical correlation observed in the '80s in real in vivo and in vitro experiments. This study is old news just the book came out recently and made system angry. Here is one example from sciencebasedmedicine.org. "I did not look at the praise or criticism of others until after I read the book, and the following represents my independent impressions. I approached the book as I do any book with scientific references: I read until I come across a statement of fact that strikes me as questionable, and then I check the references given for the statement. This immediately got me off on the wrong foot with this book. In the first chapter, I found the statement: "Heart disease can be prevented and even reversed by a healthy diet." Good doctor concluded that: "Health is more than just diet." You can trust The SkepDoc. Forget the study that took ten years and was compiled on 894 pages. She would tell you the real truth. She is a retired family physician who writes about pseudoscience and questionable medical practices, completed her internship in the Air Force (the second female ever to do so). How wrong of Dr. Campbell to say that. There are no pills to sell. He did write in the book that: "Eating foods that contain any cholesterol above 0 mg is unhealthy." Just imagine that. Dr. Campbell observed a correlation between cholesterol and heart disease back in the '80s. Very scientific and unbiased review of scienebasedmadice.org.

This kind of conflicting data made my life hard. I had to spend years of my own research because of the systematic corruption. Are you confused? Here is one statistic from the study. In Guizhou county, there was no single recorded coronary artery disease death from 246,000 men over a period of 3 years. There is nothing natural about heart disease. Number one terrorist killer in the west. Also, if you are still confused and know for sure that refined carbs like white rice are terrible and that is associated with insulin spikes and diabetes, you are right. However, wait you are wrong at the same time. You have been confused on purpose. So let do it again and look the entire picture of white rice and diabetes. When rice or grain is refined, the bran is removed. People like nice and soft bread or rice without fiber that can stick between our teeth and taste bad. However, because fiber slows down digestion and absorbs water the carbs in rice without it gets absorbed more rapidly and create unnatural insulin spike causing unnatural reaction in our body witch by compensation adapts by downregulation of insulin receptors. That is causing insulin resistance and is one of many factors that people with diabetes have to cut out of the diet. Another factor is intercellular fat that blocks insulin receptors signaling. So refined carbs and sugars cause fast digestion of large and unnatural quantities of calories.

Because we have absorption of sugar at a fast rate, we do not burn all of the calories because there are too many in the bloodstream, some will end up stored as fat. What is worse, as soon is digestion is over, and all the sugars are out of the blood we will start to feel hungry again. So lack of fiber is correlated with constant bunch eating which then causes obesity and insulin receptors downregulation. Then obesity independently causes all the bad stuff I already wrote about before, and the loop is finished. One small intervention like I do not like sticking bran in my teeth can cause a cascade of effects. A big chunk of the medical community finds that carbs are the cause of all evil and all diseases that we have today. This is base of reasoning for diets like Paleo and Atkins diet. There is no bad logic here. So far.

What is problematic is that most doctors do not read studies to the end but stick to one thing if it suits the interest of their employers. They like this kind of research if it goes along with their line of conducting business. They can sell protein powders and supplements and all the meat they can, especially if the meat is lean. You know chicken breast and maybe some with healthy fats like tuna. And all of this entire lean meat no sugar thing is just one big marketing scam. Add some bodybuilders in the picture and some fitness ladies, and there you go. You even have science to back it up. And of course a couple of good doctors to write some books.

Many people with diabetes that start to adopt this kind of diet may worsen their condition, and I will explain the whole truth and stuff they do not tell. Also, yes they know all about this but don't like to tell. For example, modern diabetes epidemic in China and Japan has been linked to white rice consumption which is another half-truth. Consequently, that is why The China Study irritates people. Rice currently feeds almost half of the world population but how can we settle much lower diabetes rates just a few decades ago when they ate even more rice? In this study for example (White rice consumption and risk of type 2 diabetes: a meta-analysis and systematic review doi: 10.1136/bmj.e1454) higher consumption of white rice was correlated with a significantly heightened chance of type 2 diabetes, particularly in Asian (Chinese and Japanese) populations. Also, this is not a small study, 352,384 participants with follow-up periods ranging from 4 to 22 years. If we analyze this statistically by total population numbers, the dose-response meta-analysis showed that for every meal per day addition of white rice intake, the relative risk of type 2 diabetes was 1.11 meaning 11% increase in risk. Today China has the same diabetes rates around 10% as the US that has around 11% despite the seven times less obesity. White rice does not appear to be correlated with obesity and heart attacks and strokes, just diabetes. However, again if we look at The China Study rural plant-based diets centered around rice were associated with a low risk of diabetes and cancer and heart disease. This 10% diabetes prevalence just happened. In the year 2000, China had one of the lowest diabetes rates in the world. This is a dramatic shift that happened in just 20 years. So what happened? Well, the same thing that happens in every country when the standard of living goes up. Meat consumption went up by an astonishing 40 percent, and rice consumption went down 30 percent. And now we have a problem. If meat consumption goes up, rice consumption goes down, and diabetes risk goes up, and at the same time, rice consumption independently is correlated with diabetes risk, what is going on? Is it just rice?

Should we eat more paleo type diet and cut all the rice right? That is what they tell us. Refined carbohydrates are correlated with diabetes and obesity. The answer is simple. What happens is that animal protein is making the rice much worse. This is one study you should go and read (Differential effect of protein and fat ingestion on blood glucose responses to high- and low-glycemic-index carbohydrates in noninsulin-dependent diabetic subjects. doi: 10.1093/ajcn/50.4.773). The date of publication was Oct 1989.

Real new medical breakthrough. Six noninsulin-dependent diabetic subjects had received meals containing 25 g carbohydrate either as potato or as spaghetti. That is the same meal as white rice. Pure white flour pasta and starch-rich low fiber potato. Then insulin response was measured, and the meals were duplicated including the bonus of 25 g protein and another one including 25 g of fat. Level of sugar in the blood and insulin responses were measured for 4h after the test meal. The addition of protein increased the insulin responses dramatically. This is a cutting-edge science to give someone sugar and protein and measure the insulin response. So there you have it. The answer. It is the holy grail of nutrition. The Protein. If we look at the chart, we would see that the addition of protein makes potato exactly two times worse. From 150 to 300.

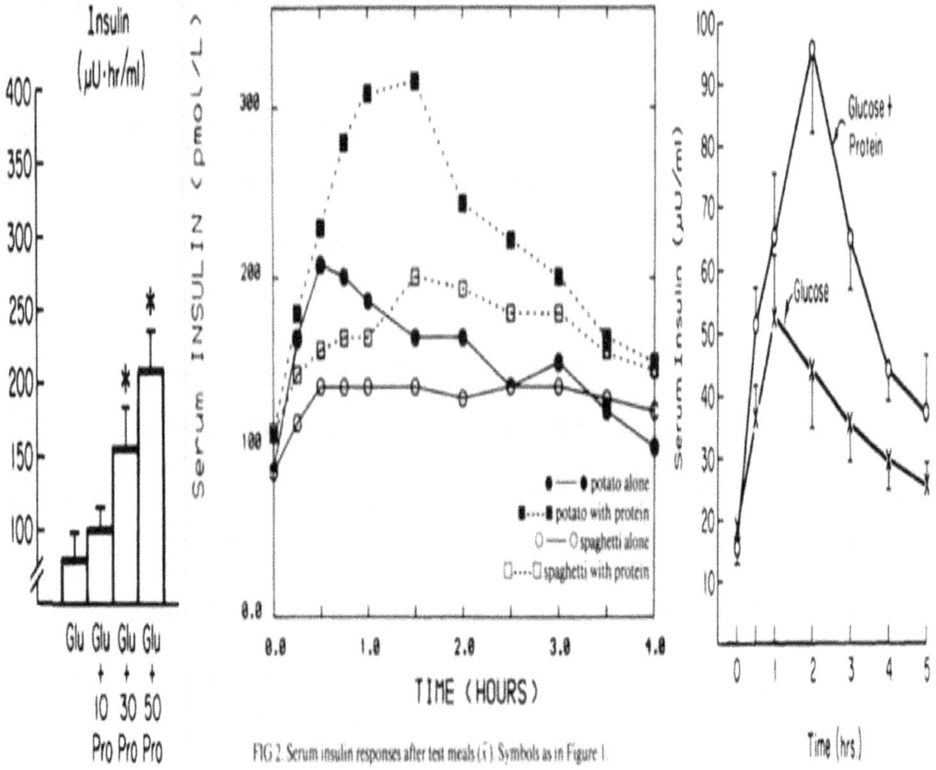

FIG 2. Serum insulin responses after test meals (1). Symbols as in Figure 1.

We can do it with sugar water too. From 50 to 100. The more meat we add, the worse it gets. When we get to 50 g of protein, we will elicit the surge of insulin that is seriously unnatural and disease-causing. Animal protein significantly potentiates the insulin secretion triggered by carbohydrate ingestion. And all along we had been told that white rice is what is causing diabetes and white flour and sugar. And that is correct partially. The real truth is more complicated. Fiber will lower insulin response like whole wheat pasta but not in the level of 100 percent. Adding meat to any starch is problematic. This combination is unnatural. It is much worse, almost two times worse for insulin response to eat roasted chicken breast with whole wheat bread then same portion of regular white flour like Pomodoro pasta with or without oil. Think about it this way. Does any other animal have regular lunch that consists of different food items? Carnivores eat only meat. Plant eaters eat only plants. What about omnivores? Do we think that bear is going to catch a fish and then don't eat it for some period until there is lunchtime so that he can bring that fish to the beehive in order to have dessert afterwards? Even combining different food items at the same meal is 100% unnatural and modern human invention. And this surge of insulin is maladaptation. I would ask this. Can we eat just meat without bread? Would we enjoy greasy sausages just by themselves? Would we enjoy just meat from burger without the buns? It is a mixture of fat and carbohydrates (sugar) that abnormally triggers dopamine signaling in our brains and many other things like in this case abnormal insulin reaction. Combining this with low fiber intake it is a recipe for disaster. Combining different food items is not a natural form of eating, but it is pleasurable so we will have to deal with it in the best way we can.

Type 2 diabetes is treatable to some extent. It is actually pretty simple. If we count out the exercise and losing weight number one would be no animal protein. Number two would be fiber. Meaning a lot of it in every meal. If you have to eat meat and have no other choice, then go ahead and eat meat. Just meat. No bread, rice or any sugar with it. Sugar meaning regular sugar or fructose or carbs in any form. No salads no nothing. Maybe some cheese. No milk. Milk has sugar or lactose in it. If you have to eat a combination of sugars and proteins before you die, then go and buy some psyllium husk or regular wheat bran and eat spoons of it after a meal. That will slow down digestion to some degree. Psyllium husk has no calories; it is 100 percent fiber. We can use it for diets if we want to bulk meals in the stomach to give us more saturation but it tastes like cardboard that is liquid. Number three would be resistant starch meaning beans. If you do not like flatulence, then go and stick the needle. Also, if you eat sausages with lots of bread and lots of alcohol you are probably done deal if you have diabetes in the family. When we see the numbers that 1 in 10 people have diabetes, it is an understatement. The actual number is 1 in 3 people in developed countries; just they might not know it because they do not have visible symptoms and insulin resistance is in the range that is known as pre-diabetes. Pre-diabetes is a disease just by itself and would also cause in the long run some adverse effects. It escalates to full-blown diabetes in 1 in 10 cases. CDC estimates that this numbers will still grow primarily on the global scale as the industrialization of the undeveloped regions of the world is taking place. If you have pre-diabetes, the long-term damage especially to your heart, blood vessels and kidneys may already be starting. This is what regular medical industry like Mayo Clinic has to say about it: "The exact cause of pre-diabetes is unknown. However, family history and genetics appear to play an important role. Inactivity and excess fat especially abdominal fat also seem to be important factors." Yes, yes, they are lying. They are always telling half-truths. Genetics is not the culprit. Maladaptation is. I know, and they know, and we all know what causes diabetes. Type 2 at least and to a great extent even type 1. Type 1 is also maladaptation. In the real world without insulin, an example would be human civilization just 200 years ago, having type 1 diabetes is an instant death sentence and to great extend type 2 also. Babies born with it and people who got it would most likely die, and their genes would be selected against. Type 1 diabetes is still a modern disease. To be fair for Mayo Clinic maybe they cannot say it blatantly because of the corruption. What they will do at least is tell us this: "Eating red meat and processed meat, and drinking sugar-sweetened beverages, is associated with a higher risk of pre-diabetes. A diet high in fruits, vegetables, nuts, seeds, whole grains, and olive oil is associated with a lower risk of pre-diabetes." Their prevention guide includes healthy foods, physical activity, losing excess pounds and control of blood pressure and cholesterol because: "Research indicates that prediabetes is often associated with unrecognized heart attacks and can damage your kidneys, even if you have not progressed to type 2 diabetes." What research and how? For average men out there what is a connection between diabetes and heart attack? Just obey them, right. Half-truths. If we interpret the meaning between the lines, we would see what they are saying. Problem is most people do not. At the end of the day, meat is just meat. The composition is the same if not identical no matter if it is white or red. Some may have more fat some less, but all of them will act the same. Mayo will include other risk factors like weight, inactivity and genetic predisposition. Why olive oil, not other oils? Because olive oil is a predominantly monosaturated form of oil that will not oxidize at the same level as polyunsaturated oil. Result of oxidation would be oxidative inflammation, meaning turning itself into rancid oil quickly. Saturated oil or in other word fat, oxidize even slower than monosaturated. However, saturated fat is exactly what causes diabetes along with animal protein. Two of them both come in the same product, the meat. The overall inflammation plays the role, meaning a low level of chronic inflammation will worsen your condition and condition of all western diseases, and that comes along with meat and toxins and lack of antioxidants. It all comes as a package with a single cause of maladaptation to the modern diet. When they talk about fat all the time is not just dietary fat it is also abdominal fat. Our own fat is also saturated. Abdominal fat worsens the condition because of something that is known as the spillover effect. FFA or Free Fatty Acids or just fat in bloodstream results in inflammation naturally. When fat is broken down there are toxic byproducts and oxidative stress which will block insulin receptor pathway and lead to insulin resistance in the muscle (Role of insulin in the pathogenesis of free fatty acid-induced insulin resistance in skeletal muscle. Endocr Metab Immune Disord Drug Targets. 2007 Mar;7(1):65-74). As the level of fat in bloodstream rises the ability of the body to clear sugar drops. I want to write this again. As the level of fat in bloodstream rises the ability of the body to clear sugar drops (How free fatty acids inhibit glucose utilization in human skeletal muscle. News Physiol Sci. 2004 Jun;19:92-6.). No big science here, nothing secret. The problem is that we are not designed to cope with sizeable saturated fat intake at the single sitting like carnivorous animals. They can eat to the extreme and we cannot. With the high amount of calories coming from meat and with much-saturated fat that is in there too and even worse, starch without fiber with animal protein combination the entire situation is aggravated. One other thing also aggravates all of this. Fat does not need to come from food it also comes from our own deposits. When we gain weight the number of fat cells does not rise. We have a constant number of them. What happens is that they just became larger with more fat in them.

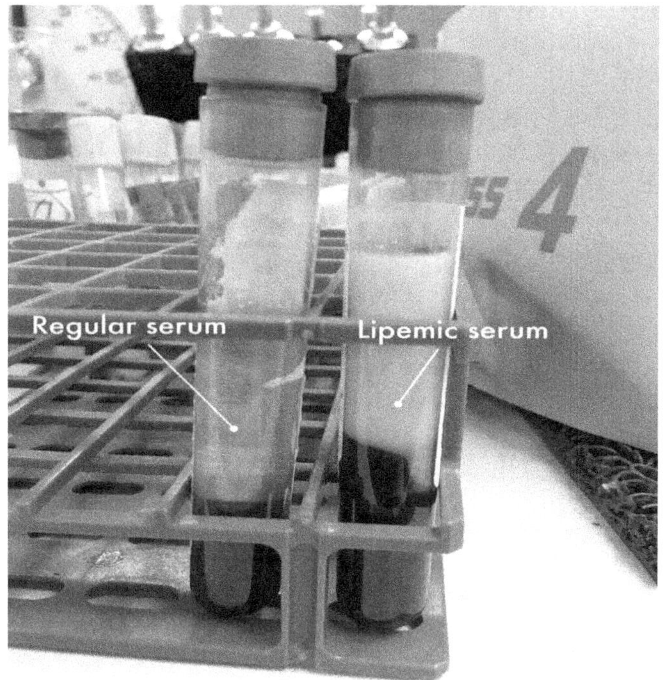

How large could a fat cells get? They can but at one point they will become bloated and will start to spill the fat back into the bloodstream even if there is no need for it. Because of the spillover effect obese person will have a higher fat concentration not just around their body but in the bloodstream too and will worsen the aggravation even more for diabetes and different types of other diseases. Because this fat cannot be adequately stored and there is no need for it, it will loge itself in different cells including muscle cells, stick itself to arteries, it will make blood more ticker with less fluidity and so on.

We are meant to cope well with utilizing fat, it is essential for life, but even this has a crossing line. This is why we have to fast for 9 to 12 hours before the blood test profile is to be taken. This will eliminate any effects of a recent meal on blood lipids such as cholesterol and triglycerides. In obesity blood tests are lipemic to some degree all the time, leading to insulin resistance and promoting type 2 diabetes. If we put people on a low carb high-fat diet, fats build up in their muscles in just two hours compared to a low-fat diet (Effects of intravenous and dietary lipid challenge on intramyocellular lipid content and the relation with insulin sensitivity in humans. Diabetes. 2001 Nov;50(11):2579-84). Fat meaning saturated fat without any fibers to slow down digestion meaning animal protein. Just hours after meat consumption our bodies have a problem using insulin. I will write this again. Just hours after meat consumption our bodies have a problem using insulin. High fat and protein paleo, Atkins type keto diets are not suited for pre-diabetics. None of the animal products are. I am putting all of this citations because this irritates industry so much. Even institutions like Mayo Clinic go with the line. I do not live from medicine. I can write whatever I want to write, and you can go and do your own research, so I do not care. Consult your regular MD before doing any changes to your lifestyle. I had pre-diabetes myself, and I had diabetes type 2 in the family. I had numerous high-level specialist telling me to eat low-fat meat and fish and to avoid sugar and carbs like rice. This is one of many topics that forced me into research of my own. When I mention something like this (Red meat consumption and risk of type 2 diabetes: 3 cohorts of US adults and an updated meta-analysis. Am J Clin Nutr. 2011 Oct;94(4):1088-96) where investigators discovered that for each 3.5 ounces of red meat eaten daily, diabetes chance rose 10% and for each 1.75 ounces of processed red meat eaten daily (about one packaged hot dog), the risk increased 51%, they didn't like it. There are the only ones that have authority on what is truth and who are we? I might don't know as much, but I think that at least I might not be an idiot. I write what I know.

Carbohydrates are not bad. They will not make us fat and sick. They do not turn to sugar and make us get diabetes. It is precisely the opposite. We are living in the reality of inversion. In Japan word for cooked rice gohan also means meal. The word for breakfast as gohan is morning rice. In China word for rice also means food. Chinese don't ask: "How are you?". They ask: "Have you had your rice today?", as an expression. In India the situation is similar. It is the first food the bride offers her husband which is better than in Indonesia where there is no marriage until the bride is able to prepare the rice skillfully. Where is obesity there, where is diabetes, where is cancer, stroke or heart disease? These countries may have cholera or some other infectious disease problem, but that is a consequence of low sanitation. They do not have diabetes. The fact that type 2 diabetes mostly preventable disease has reached such a high level is a humiliation to the medical community.

What about type 1? In type 1 there is no insulin resistance, but pancreas or more specific cells named beta cells are damaged. These cells in normal conditions produce insulin but because they are dead or damaged they do not. By the age of 20, we have all the beta cells we would because they do not regenerate like liver cells for example. If we lose them, it is for good. On autopsy studies with people who had diabetes type 2, they found that by the time type 2 diabetes is diagnosed beta cells numbers are down to around 50 percent and that number decreases even more as life progresses. So besides insulin resistance, there are some form of pre-diabetes of type 1 in pre-diabetes of type 2 individuals to some extent. What kills them, these beta insulin-producing cells? The answer is the same. Fat. To be more precise only the saturated fat, not vegetable oil. We can even do it directly in a Petri dish. Take some beta cells and put fat on top of them, they suck it up and die (Lipotoxicity: effects of dietary saturated and trans fatty acids. doi:10.1155/2013/137579). Fatty acid derivate interferes with the function of beta cells and ultimately lead to their death through lipoapoptosis. Lipo meaning fat, Greek (lípos, animal fat) and apoptosis meaning process of programmed cell death. Alternatively, just fat kills them. In the above paper, they concluded it is because all the inflammation that comes along with animal fat. Fatty acids are involved in several inflammatory pathways, contributing to chronic inflammation, disease progression, cancer, allergy, hypertension, atherosclerosis, and heart hypertrophy as well as other metabolic and degenerative diseases. As a consequence, lipotoxicity may occur in several target organs including the pancreas. It can happen by direct effects, represented by inflammation pathways, and through indirect effects, including an essential alteration in the gut microbiota associated with endotoxemia. It feeds all the bad bacteria in the gut that will multiply exponentially and then secrete toxins into the bloodstream. As a consequence, the immune system response will be triggered causing inflammation and DNA damage. Interactions between these pathways may perpetuate a feedback process that exacerbates an inflammatory state. Also, I will add to this that when combined with inflammatory nutrient deprived diet that comes when we eat animal protein with fat and not plant protein that comes with antioxidants, there are no nutrients to stop the inflammation. Don't get me wrong lipotoxicity will happen even if we stuff ourself with kale but lacking anti-inflammatory, antioxidant nutrient-rich food will add salt to the injury. In this paper, they did experiment to see just how much beta cells die with lipotoxicity (Death protein 5 and p53-upregulated modulator of apoptosis mediate the endoplasmic reticulum stress-mitochondrial dialog triggering lipotoxic rodent and human ß-cell apoptosis. doi: 10.2337/db12-0123.).

I deliberately want to put the names of papers in this way for you to read because I want you to be accustomed to reading them. Medical branch has their secret language, and they have a strict hierarchy like an army with different titles and colors and stuff like that. The underline message is that they are so smart and so important and so much smarter than us so don't ask questions and most importantly of all, do as told. Do not do anything they do not approve or you are going to die. What happens, in reality, is that when you are literary about to die, and they give you month or two to live then people and only then start to do their own thinking, and by that time it is already too late. So go ahead and read papers yourself there is no mystery there after learning some basics of the mystery language we will be able to do it with no problem. Let's do some mystery language discovery.

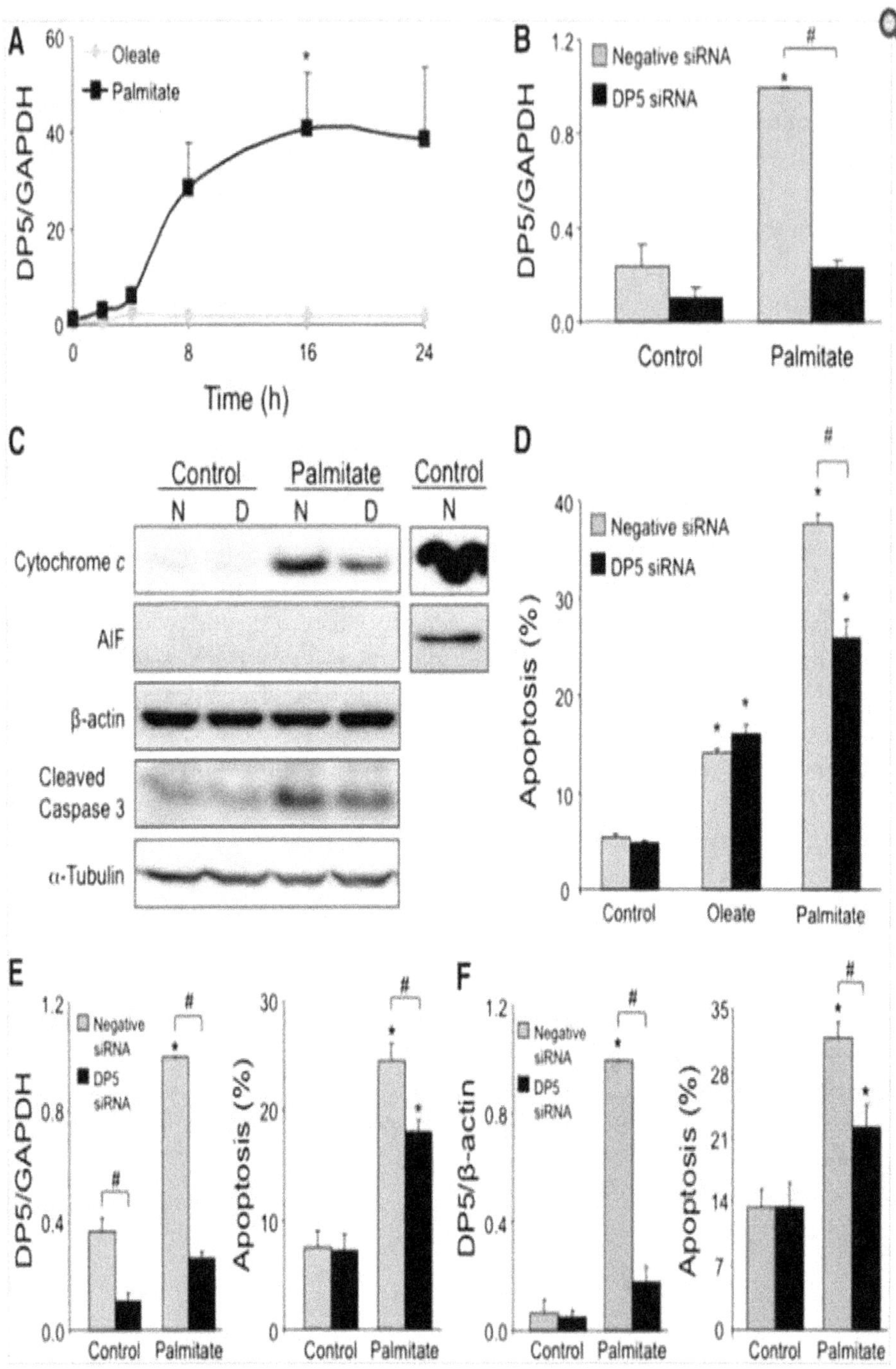

Palmitate-induced *DP5* expression contributes to β-cell death. *A*: Time-course analysis of *DP5* mRNA expression in oleate- or p

Oleate is fat in nuts and olives, and palmitate is fat in saturated fat of just fat from animals. We know what beta cell is and we know that apoptosis means death so do your own analysis of the chart from this mystery language study. If you just not into it then look at chart A, and you will see the difference in "Palmitate-induced DP5 expression contribution to ß-cell apoptosis" or just in normal language how much animal fat kills insulin-producing cells. Also, it is not just fat; cholesterol does it independently as result of oxidative stress or ROS (reactive oxygen species) formation (Fatty acids and glucolipotoxicity in the pathogenesis of Type 2 diabetes. doi: 10.1042/BST0360348).

What causes diabetes? At least type 2 is consumption of a hypercaloric diet rich in animal protein (saturated fat) in individuals that have more of genetic predisposition to it. Aggravation of disease is infused with combination and consumption of animal protein and carbohydrates at a single sitting. How many people know this? Not even dietician specialist will tell you this. Are you still confused? I will mention one more study (High-carbohydrate, high-fiber diets for insulin-treated men with diabetes mellitus. Am J Clin Nutr. 1979 Nov;32(11):2312-21). It was done back in 1979. To exclude weight loss from the positive impact on blood sugar levels they had to weight subjects every day and force them to eat more in many occasions. At the end of the study, there were no significant alterations in body weight despite restriction in animal product consumption. Weight loss was excluded as a possible influential factor. They were restricted in meat, dairy, eggs, and junk and were allowed to eat whole food plant based diet only. The result was as follows: average insulin dose was reduced from 26 units/day on the control diets to 11. That is a 65% reduction and half of the people with diabetes were off the insulin completely. Many of these subjects were on diabetic medications for as long as 20 years. After years on medication injecting 26 units of insulin a day on average, half of them were able to get off completely with plant-based diet. Imagine that.

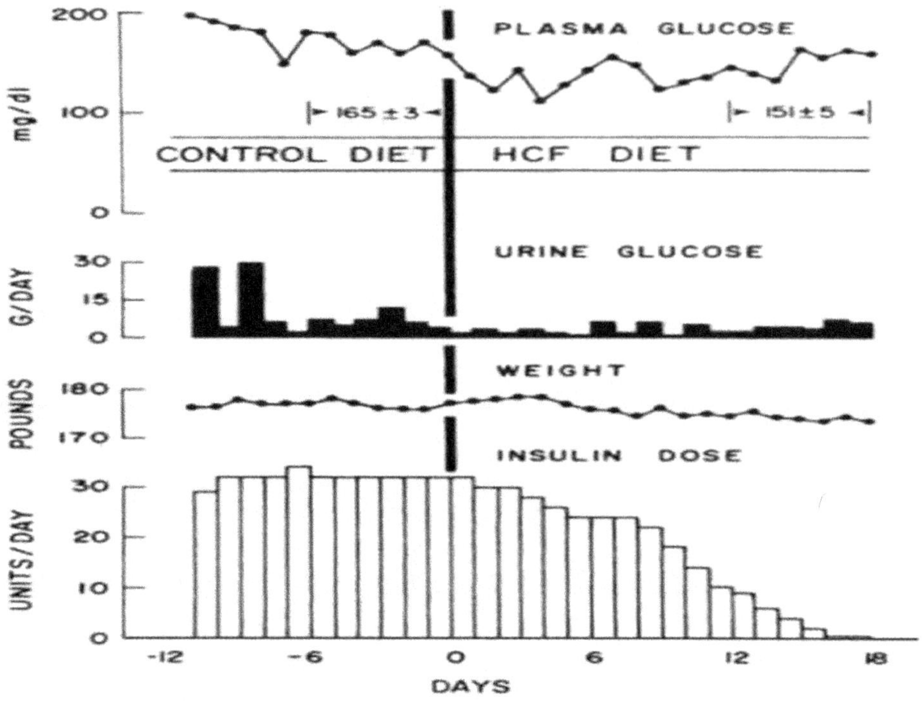

You are injecting yourself for 20 years with no cure, and then some "stupid" vegan diet gets you off insulin. What do you think, how much time did it take for a diet to work? Year or two, or a couple of months? It took 16 days. You have diabetes for 20 years injecting 26 units of insulin a day, and then 16 days later you are free. Why has nobody ever told you about this study? Why has nobody ever told you about a plant-based diet? There is the chart above with results for patient number 15. He was having 32 units of insulin on the control diet and then 16 days later, zero. Is this just a fluke? It is all maybe just indication of control of information and corruption on the systematic scale. I can only compare medical schools of today with cigarettes companies of the past. Cigarettes companies did hire doctors to brand their products as a health promoting habit. Back in the day when smoking was normal.

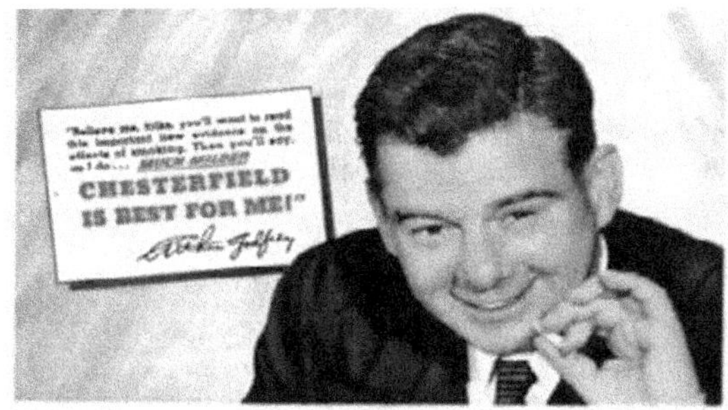
"Believe me, folks, you'll want to read this important new evidence on the effects of smoking. Then you'll say, as I do... MUCH MILDER
CHESTERFIELD
IS BEST FOR ME!"
NOW...Scientific Evidence
on Effects of Smoking!
A MEDICAL SPECIALIST is making regular bi-monthly examinations of a group of people from various walks of life. 45 percent of this group have smoked Chesterfield for an average of over ten years.
After ten months, the medical specialist reports that he observed....
no adverse effects on the nose, throat and sinuses of the group from smoking Chesterfield.
MUCH MILDER
CHESTERFIELD
IS BEST FOR YOU
First and Only Premium Quality Cigarette in Both Regular and King-Size
Chesterfield
CIGARETTES
Chesterfield
KING-SIZE
CIGARETTES
APRIL 1953

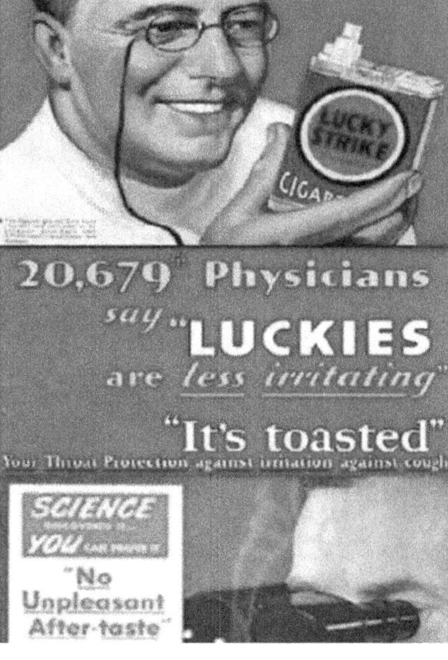
LUCKY STRIKE
CIGAR
20,679 Physicians
say "LUCKIES
are less irritating"
"It's toasted"
Your Throat Protection against irritation against cough
SCIENCE
YOU
"No
Unpleasant
After-taste"

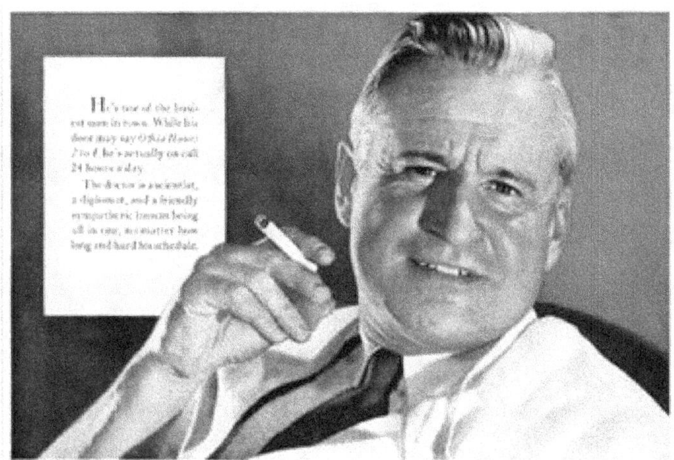
According to a recent Nationwide survey:
MORE DOCTORS SMOKE CAMELS
THAN ANY OTHER CIGARETTE
CAMEL
CAMELS Costlier Tobaccos
Your "T-Zone" Will Tell You...
T for Taste...
T for Throat...

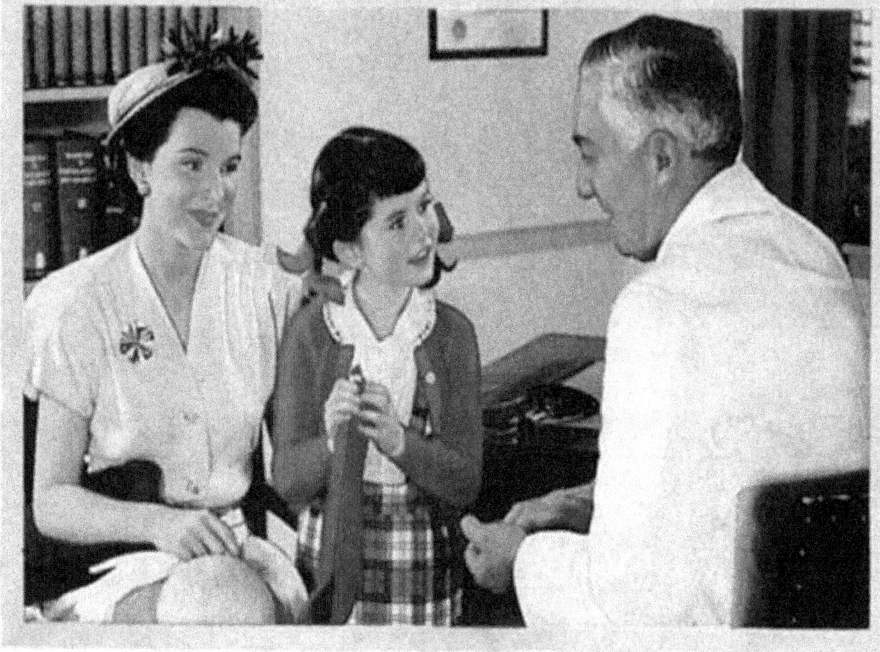

According to a recent Nationwide survey:

More Doctors smoke Camels
than any other cigarette!

NOT ONE but three outstanding independent research organizations conducted this survey. And they asked not just a few thousand, but 113,597, doctors from coast to coast to name the cigarette they themselves preferred to smoke.

Answers came in by the thousands... from general physicians, diagnosticians, surgeons, nose and throat specialists too. The most-named brand was Camel.

If you are not now smoking Camels, try them. Let your "T-Zone" tell you (see right).

R. J. Reynolds Tobacco Co., Winston-Salem, N. C.

CAMELS *Costlier Tobaccos*

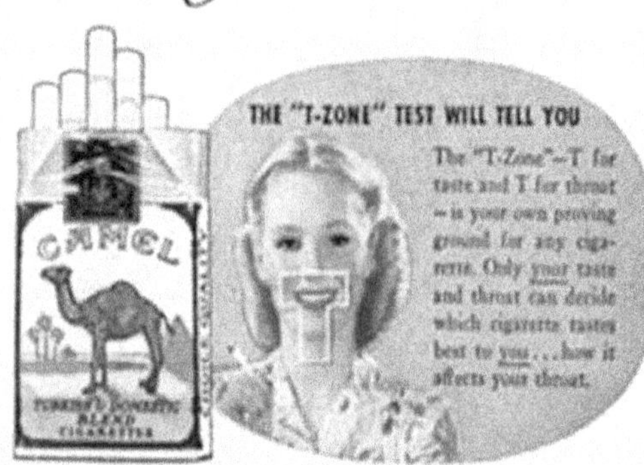

In the 40s and in times before that, the pinch line of MD's was that nicotine kills microbes and then smoking is somehow protective against tuberculosis. In the world, without antibiotics, it is strong fear to manipulate, and now there is even filter in there to filter out all the bad stuff. Did you hear "20,679 physicians say 'Luckies are less irritating," See that little girl on the picture? "She is going to grow a 100 years old. A whole decade longer than her mother and good 20 years longer than her grandmother." Not only that but she will be much healthier too. Thank medical science for that. In reality, she will not go to even '80s as her granny did. She will have a heart attack, diabetes, stroke or cancer maybe even in her 30s. For regular Joe out there who is not emotionally damaged it would be a hard time resisting this type of propaganda. It took more than 50 years to prove that inhaling smoke might not be a good idea. After the industrial revolution everything was capitalized, including medicine, turned upside down and entire way of life was denatured. Most of the medical students are naive. They think that science they learn in the college is truthful and most of them start to integrate the belief system into their ego. It is an organization like an army or any other hierarchical structure where brainwashing of cadets takes place. If MD starts to deviate from accepted science his job is on the line. Usually they will have much more patients in a day then they should by design, so that they would not have much time for every single patient and will go assembly line style of learned responses. Symptoms drugs, symptoms drugs and so on. No real help there. This is just a business model. If you have any doubts, then ask this question. Why is not nutrition taught in medical schools? The reason is industrialization, corruption, and capitalization. In rural China or other places that are still poor they do not suffer from modern diseases, but also they do not give most of their income on good service of modern medicine. Even in religious groups who have a rigid lifestyle the situation is similar like for example, the Adventist study showed. Adventist Health Studies (AHS) is a group of long-term studies done by Loma Linda University. They do this studies to see if there is any link between lifestyle and mortality and diseases of Seventh-day Adventists. In the most recent study that is still being conducted, AHS-2, around 100,000 church members are enrolled from both the US and Canada. For more than 100 years the Seventh-day Adventist Church had been promoting health behaviors that had become the regular part of daily living. These include not smoking, eating a plant-based diet, regular exercise and maintaining healthy body weight. Seventh-day Adventists do have a measurable lower risk than other Americans for most of the western diseases. The connection is based like in other rural parts of undeveloped countries of the world on dietary habits. Also, some part on exercise. Over the past 40 years, two Adventist health studies have been conducted involving 22,940 and 34,000 Californian Adventists.

The first significant study of Adventists started in 1958 and became known as the Adventist Mortality Study. It involved an intensive 5-year follow-up with a more informal 25-year follow-up. By comparing all causes of death Adventist men had a mortality rate of 66% and Adventist women had a rate of 88%. Overall mortality of cancer compared to their counterparts in the American Cancer Society was 60% for Adventist men and 76% for Adventist women. America is 100% baseline, so 60% meaning 40% lower rates. Lung cancer was 21 percent, meaning 80% lower rates, colorectal cancer deaths were 62 percent. Breast cancer death rates for Adventist women were 85 percent; prostate cancer death rates for Adventist men were 92 percent. Death due to coronary disease among Adventist men was 66%; for Adventist women, it was 98%. The stroke death rates for Adventist men were 72%; Adventist women 82%. We have to understand that the study was done back in the 60s.

Why is this important? Because they eat a plant-based diet for religious reasons not necessarily for scientific reasons. They eat a diet that is vegan but not necessarily optimized. Sugar is vegan, so is oil, salt and chips and bunch of other junk. Eating plant-based diet essentially means little if we don't know precisely why we eat or not eat something. Vegans who go into this kind of lifestyle for moral reasons may end up in worse health condition then before they consumed many animal products if they do not know precisely what they are doing. Adventist as a group are more educated than the rest of the Californians, and they did have to calculate that into the study. The more education we have the greater the chance is that we will go more to healthier food choices independently from any other factor. Leonardo da Vinci, for example, had eaten an ovo-lacto-vegetarian diet just by his conviction of human anatomy. He did cut corpses for science. In the end, this rates can be much better, and this study was done back in the 60s. The situation is worse today for the average American with skyrocketing obesity, diabetes and so on. Current study Adventist Health Study 2 (AHS-2) which began in 2002 also had some sub-studies later. For example, (Vegetarian Dietary Patterns and Mortality in Adventist Health Study 2 JAMA Intern Med. 2013 Jul 8; 173(13): 1230–1238) and (Vegetarian diets and incidence of diabetes in the Adventist Health Study-2 Nutr Metab Cardiovasc Dis. 2013 Apr;23(4):292-9). They concluded that: "Vegetarian diets are associated with lower all-cause mortality and with some reductions in cause-specific mortality." The more plan based we go, the more all-cause and cause-specific mortality drops and not just that. We might live ten years longer or 15, it does not matter. What matter is that we would avoid most of the diseases of affluence which include osteoporosis, type 2 diabetes, cardiovascular disease, obesity, breast cancer, colorectal cancer and most of the other cancers, acne, gout, depression, and diseases related to vitamin and mineral deficiencies to many to count and all the prescription drugs side effects. Standard American meat-eating diet is so healthy that with all the calories and complete animal proteins and eggs and dairy, 92% people eating it are potassium deficient, 57% deficient in magnesium, more than 80 percent deficient in vitamin E. I don't even want to talk about non-essential minerals, antioxidants, phytochemicals, iodine, vitamin D, selenium and so on. Minimal recommended values are in many cases deliberately low. Like, for example, RDA for iodine. This story is the story of quality of life. Treatment is expensive. Drug addicts are best customers. Eventually, they will spend all of their money just to keep their habit. In this case, it is supernormal stimuli in the form of food. These diseases of affluence have vastly increased in prevalence since the end of World War 2 and will continue to increase as the standard of living and meat consumption skyrocket worldwide. They have already been increasing in prevalence even before WW2 in the most developed countries in the world. For instance, in the middle of the last century in England, cardiovascular diseases have already reached a point of 5 to 10 percent of mortality rate. England has been keeping mortality statistics for a very long time. They first started back in 1665. The mortality rate for cardiovascular disease was practically unknown at the beginning of the 20th century and then started to increase in the 1920s. From this study where they analyzed the historical progression of heart disease rate in England, we can see the charts and the rate of expansion (Ryle JA, Russell WT. The natural history of coronary disease; a clinical and epidemiological study. Br Heart J. 1949;11(4):370-89).

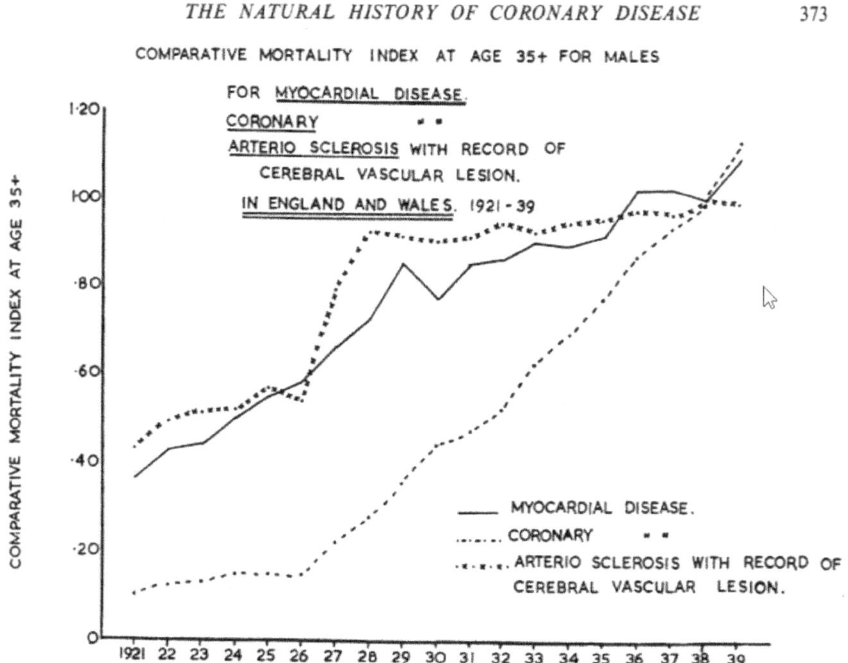

FIG. 1.—Comparative mortality index at age 35+ for males for myocardial disease, coronary disease, and arterio-sclerosis with record of cerebral vascular lesion, in England and Wales 1921–39.

It was well known to the medical community what is going on even back then. Nathan Pritikin cured heart disease by a regimen of diet decades ago, followed by Dr. Dean Ornish and then Dr. Caldwell Esselstyn at the Cleveland Clinic. In my view, there is nothing that will change this situation on a global scale. I can write 20 books, there can be 1000 other ones, and that will probably mean nothing. Drugs are drugs, and drug addicts usually do not like rehab. However, if we do a diet shift then what can we expect realistically?

If we look at average Adventist that is health-conscious among other Adventist, meaning the ones that avoid junk and exercise, they live 87 years for man and 89 years for a woman at average. That is even higher than Okinawa Japanese in the past. Okinawa is also one good example if we want to see what dietary shift can do. Traditional Okinawa diet was plant-based. They will eat a small amount of fish or pork or other meat, but that is in a range of a couple of percent. Meaning maybe once or twice a month. Not once or twice a week. Once or twice a month. Rest of it is plant-based. Traditional Japanese diet usually includes large quantities of rice. Traditional Okinawa diet is not based on rice but instead on the purple sweet potato. Back in 1950 from 1262 grams of all food consumed, sweet potato made up 849 grams or 69% of total calories. Rice was 12 %, grains 7%, 6% legumes meaning soy and other beans and that is it. Fish is around 1 %, pork and other meat less than 1%, eggs less than 1%, dairy is less than 1%. Asian populations are lactose intolerant. This diet is as same as any other "incomplete" poor people diet. This is essentially the same as rural China or any other starch-based diet influenced by poverty just in their case they had sweet potatoes. No complete protein high fat keto diet there. We can see what they used to eat just by looking at US National Archives because US army run Okinawa island until 1972. However, if we ask some of the corporate doctors about this they cannot deny it.

What is their exit strategy? Take a pause in reading and think of one for yourself. If you like your half million dollars annually, what will your response be? If you ask them, they will again tell you half-truths and direct lies. Here is one example from Dr. Axe whose motto is: "Food is medicine." He has a book "The Real food diet" and sells supplements like "Dr. Axe Multi Collagen Protein." Collagen, by the way, is a globular protein that does not pass into the bloodstream undigested same as any other protein. It gets digested (broken down) to individual amino acids again as any other globular proteins do and I can pretty much be confident that most of you out there do not have any amino acid deficiencies what so ever. We can only increase or try to increase collagen production by our own body indigenously. Eating collagen is like eating anything else. So what will they say? If they cannot avoid it, then they will acknowledge it by saying that Okinawans do eat healthy. A diet full of antioxidants and carotenoids and: "Though the Okinawa diet does allow for meat and seafood, it does so in small, limited quantities. Barring festivals or special occasions, stick to a mostly plant-based diet. We can replicate this at home by eating high-quality meats and seafood, like grass-fed beef, bison meat and wild-caught seafood like salmon. Enjoying these foods just a few times a week or on special occasions means we will enjoy the benefits of healthy fats, like reducing inflammation, controlling cholesterol and reducing our risk for heart disease, while keeping calories in check."

Let's do some math. If we eat meat two times a week and of course Dr. Axe will say that we can eat meat every day if it is grass-fed beef. However, if we eat meat two times a week that is eight times a month and that is 10% of meals and little less than 10% of calories. To get to 1 % of real Okinawa diet, it is only once a month. Eating 10% makes it ok in the subconscious mind, and you go right back to eating it every day. It is not meat that is a culprit, that is the underlying message. It is bad quality of meat. So meat is good if it is grass-fed beef and bison and wild caught salmon. You see now how information gets twisted. Moreover, then doctors who like their salaries like Dr. Axe will outline the dangers of low-fat dairy, including the fact that it is often full of added sugar including the fact that pasteurization method destroys a lot of the helpful enzymes and vitamins. When you start to think that he is just against any saturated fat and would recommend you not to consume milk at all, he will recommend choosing full-fat raw milk and raw dairy products which are of course completely different. He recommends low fat meat and high full-fat dairy, what? What is high-quality meat? What he means if it is not lean protein? Maybe just organic? And then he will tell you to avoid soy because of all phytoestrogens, which mimic the hormone estrogen in your body which is another half-truth. That is entirely false actually. Soy is just problematic as a cheap alternative for people who want for some unknown reason to eat high protein plant-based diet. Most of the estrogen around 80 percent, comes from dairy in standard American diet. That is full blown animal estrogen. Consequently, soy must go. What you do not know is that estrogen in soy is tens of times less potent than estradiol and actually lowers the risk of breast cancer acting like estrogen receptor blocking agent in the body. Basically the same thing as Nolvadex (Tamoxifen). It is not full-blown estradiol like in raw dairy products that Dr. Axe will recommend. Do we understand now how manipulation works?

Dr. Axe concludes that the Okinawa diet is not a magic cure, you heard it wrong. We should stick with quality meats over quantity and reducing grains. That will: "Have a positive impact on your health. Additionally, reducing your family's meat and seafood intake lessens the load on your wallet, making products that might normally be a stretch more budget-friendly", (like grass-fed beef). Reducing grains that are the starch source as same as sweet potato and we are talking here about Okinawa diet. Also, for blood sugar control "food is medicine" doctor will recommend some of the best protein foods like wild fish such as salmon, and I will add here, while you still can. Around 90 percent of fish is gone. All of the large fish both open ocean species including marlin, swordfish, tuna and the large groundwater fish such as flounder, skates, cod, and halibut, are gone according to research published in scientific journal Nature. Moreover, of course, raw dairy products (including raw cheeses, yogurt, and kefir), free-range eggs, pasture-raised poultry, and grass-fed beef or lamb. This is just standard American diet with organic products that won't do anything to improve your health. You will be just more confused, and that is precisely what bro doctors do and what their job is. If you wonder little off from the flock, they will still catch you. Moreover, all of these doctors marketing shows on TV, midnight talks and all of it. To be fair many of these people who go through the medical school are scared for their future and do what needs to be done. They might end up themselves confused, and they might actually believe they are doing good not realizing the scope of the corruption.

I do not use words lightly. It is corruption on a systematic scale. In 2013 for people with diabetes average costs were \$14,999 in the U.S. annually. For patients covered by insurance typical out of pocket cost for prescription drug copay will be in a range of ten to fifty dollars depending on the drug regimen. For multiple drug regiments, copays can total more than 200\$. For patients without health insurance for a multidrug regiment cost can range from 200 to 500 dollars a month. Even if you have copays that don't mean that drug companies do not get their money it just means you paid it from insurance, they do not care. Many countries have adopted universal health care. That is where the government pays for healthcare, just like it pays for defense and education. It is like expanding Medicare or Medicaid to everyone. They get their money in these countries too but from the government. They do not care. They even prefer governmental model because corruption is still there. Cost of manufacturing these chemicals is around zero. For you, that needs them the price is going to be substantial. As much as companies calculate that is the upper limit that they can charge. Didn't you hear it? It is all because of research and development. You remember all these commercials (regularly to overpriced brand-name pills) with a message: "Ask your doctor?" Well, don't be shy. Do exactly that and ask your doctor just how much that new prescription will cost and go generic from India as much as you possibly can before you do all the lifestyle alterations you possibly can. And don't take: "I do not know", for an answer. He knows exactly. He or she is a professional liar. Most of the stuff you need probably you would not be able to find cheap so \$500 or even higher for a month for a multi-drug regimen just from people with diabetes without pricing all the other operations and supplements and all other products. It is a nice margin for spreading the corruption.

It all began more than 100 years ago. We will analyze the history in part 2 of the book series. When the economy of the U.S. or any other developed country in the world go to recession and unemployment start to rise many of the regular people end up without medications. In developing countries, a big part of populations is without medications all the time. These companies do their business globally, so they do not care. Stockholders are mostly secret but mostly connected to international banking cartel and to some extent to other big industries. The scope is big. Do your research and whatever truth you find is yours. What they do not count is that most of the people now have uncensored internet. Well at least for the time being. Where ever we look around the world we see the same story. Okinawans had low levels of chronic diseases. Past tense. The situation is different now. They had 12 times less heart attack deaths, three to seven time less cancer depend on which type, no diabetes, no obesity. There was also a cultural norm not to overeat (hara hachi-bu), so they tend to eat fewer calories overall. They were in a state of caloric restriction to some point, not in a state of starvation big difference. Current demographic shows that their longevity is a thing of the past. Saturated fat tripled, protein doubled, cholesterol skyrocketed and all other things that come along when we start to eat KFC. It can be even seen on family pictures. Old grandparents still going slim and strong eating traditional style with their grandchildren who are obese at a young age and like to play video games, watch anime and eat meat and sugar and fat. They are now full of calories and nutrient deficient as much as the rest of the developed world. In two generations they went from leanest of Japanese people to the ones with highest BMI's. There is movement from public health professionals in Okinawa now to try to get young Okinawans to eat traditional Okinawa way. Without much of the success, I will add. Everywhere we look it is the same picture.

Even the good old healthy Mediterranean diet. Marketed as a wonder of olive oil that had nothing to do with oil of any sort what so ever except in the measure that it can replace even worse choices like regular saturated fat like butter and lard. That is precisely how even father of the Mediterranean diet saw it (A Keys. Olive oil and coronary heart disease. Lancet. 1987 Apr 25;1(8539):983-4). When you go to pubmed.gov and search for a Mediterranean diet, there are about 5000 results. Mediterranean diet is many diets in a lot of different countries. It can be Morocco or Greek or Spain or Italy or some other place. However, when we talk about Mediterranean diet what is implied is the diet in the island of Crete in the post World War 2 era. Also, what comes next is a big question: Why was heart disease rare in the Mediterranean? Meaning on the island of Crete after WW2. In 1948 after the war and socioeconomic collapse, the government of Greece was concern about malnutrition and health status of their citizens. They decided to invite the Rockefeller Foundation with the goal of undertaking an epidemiological study on the island of Crete. In 1952 impressed by low rates of heart disease Ancel Keys, the same scientist that was in charge of the Minnesota Starvation Experiment, noted the connection after researching the data between fat and especially saturated fat and heart disease. Although at that time he did not see cholesterol as the problem because it would mean the animal products are the guilty one. The connection between dietary fat and heart disease was observed even earlier in 1930's and was influential on Keys work, but data from Crete made him wrote a paper about it in 1953 and made public addresses. The famous Seven Country Study was to begin five years later in 1958 to investigate Keys concerns. By 1960s it was common belief that saturated fat contributes to heart disease. Diet of people on the island of Crete was a catalyst for this research later on. In 1970 the Seven Country Study was presented for the first time. Now Keys lived to 100 himself and at the time was not much of the radical as cholesterol confusionists would like you to believe. He recommended eating less fat, meaning fat in meat and fat in general like eggs (or at least yolks) and dairy products and instead of eating more fish and chicken. He considered fruits and vegetables to be just the complement food, and he had cholesterol of around 200. That number is not healthy by a long shot, but he did live to 100. The problem was that he was a doctor from the same system as any other doctor. Arteriosclerosis does not usually happen in age like cholesterol confusionists would like us to believe because of all of the stressful blood flow.

Arteriosclerosis is a disease, not the aging process. We can go and look at arteries and measure the blood pressure of poor people in places like Crete. Keys did not see the real truth about what was real diet on Crete. He thought it was just fat and didn't see the problem in animal protein. Animal protein correlation was overlooked even in the charts. He muddied the water by pointing just at fat. However, even that was not good enough. Even that was over the top. In 1966, George Campbell and Thomas L. Cleave published "Diabetes, Coronary Thrombosis, and the Saccharine Disease." They argued that chronic western diseases such as heart disease, peptic ulcers, diabetes, obesity are produced by one thing: "Refined carbohydrate disease." It was a never-ending story. It never stopped to this day. Everything is a lie that is confronted by opposite lie. Artificially created diet wars and confusion. It was well design strategy that didn't change a thing in 70 years except for kipping regular people in disease-causing money making an evil loop of misery. Even in current times, it is the same old manipulation story. In an 2001 for example article in Science Magazine entitled "Nutrition: The Soft Science of Dietary Fat", Gary Taubes wrote: "It is still a debatable proposition whether the consumption of saturated fats above recommended levels by anyone who's not already at high risk of heart disease will increase the likelihood of untimely death...or have hundreds of millions of dollars in trials managed to generate compelling evidence that healthy individuals can extend their lives by more than a few weeks, if that, by eating less fat."

People 70 years later think that Mediterranean diet is healthy because of olive oil. This is an excellent illustration of a half-truth. Italian restaurants market themselves as a healthy Mediterranean diet cuisine with spaghetti carbonara and alcohol. The death rate from heart disease in Crete at that time was more than 20 times, not 20 percent, 20 times less than in the US. We statistically see this data from places like rural China and Crete and Okinawa and on and on and see that these people diet is simple and similar to each other. How much of stupidity we have to have not to see the real story of what is happening. Scientists with a considerable level of education are not the stupid ones. They have six-figure annual income plus bonuses. They are the smart ones. We are not. Nutritional science is not secret deep underground military propulsion system laboratory research. There are no real debates in the field of nutrition, only purposely created real confusion.

So what did they eat at the island of Crete in World War 2 aftermath? The answer is the same. No meat, eggs, dairy. Just poor people food like fruit and vegetables, grains, nuts, legumes. Things that grow locally. In numbers, they ate more than 90% plant-based and meat, fish, dairy and eggs products combined is about 7%. They did eat some of the olive oil because olives grow in Crete but that is not the olive oil diet. Or the wine diet. There is nothing healthy about wine except grapes. We would be better off just drinking raw grape juice. If we look at Greece today what is it that we think we would find? They have the number 1 score in Europe in child obesity. The Island of Crete included. As soon as economy improves the meat, cheese, sugar, and alcohol comes in a package. And smoking too. Greece has a rate of tobacco consumption above 40%. Mediterranean diet was not a local specific Mediterranean diet like Italian cuisine or Greek cuisine or such. It was poverty diet without meat and eggs, and dairy, similar to diets in all poverty or war-stricken places and industry does not like to mention this. Heart disease was a rarity in Greece. Was. Not anymore. And even in Crete at time of war, some rich people ate "normally" meaning eating meat every day instead of once in two weeks. Heart attacks were normal for them to, unlike for the rest of common people that were struck by poverty. No one today eats real Mediterranean diet anymore. Pure Mediterranean diet of today that is predominantly plant-based is not real whole food diet. It is dominated with white flour, consumption of oil and salt and alcohol. In Crete, they did not eat refined white pasta from the factory with sauce full of extracted oil and bottles of wine. Alcohol is known breast cancer risk factor even if we disregard inflammation and toxicity. That is not a health-promoting meal. Well, that is not a health-promoting meal if we do not compare it to even worse standard American meal of today. So yes, the Mediterranean diet is healthier than the regular diet but not as healthy as real natural human diet. Whole food plant based diet.

The problem is that regular normal food is not tasty as refined full of salt and oil and sugar one so hardly anyone sticks to it. From a young age, children are given all of this chemicals we consider to be food, so we are addicted to them in childhood and have no real baseline anymore for comparison to what real human food is. That is why the poor people diet works. If we analyze the individual components of diet in Crete, we see that actually, it was not grains that were protective against heart attack. Grains, were more neutral and because they were whole food with fiber they had no effect on obesity or diabetes. Among the individual components in Mediterranean diet consumption of greens and nuts actually, have an effect on lowering cardiovascular disease risk. Vegetarians that eat nuts have a lower risk of cardiovascular disease instead of the ones that don't, and there are by now a number of studies on this topic also. Here is one (Frequency of nut consumption and mortality risk in the PREDIMED nutrition intervention trial BMC Med. 2013 Jul 16;11:164) with the conclusion: "Increased frequency of nut consumption was associated with a significantly reduced risk of mortality in a Mediterranean population at high cardiovascular risk." Nuts have high-oil content but also high fiber content, so the oil is not immediately absorbed like fat from meat or refined oil and unlike meat or oil nuts are rich in antioxidants and other phytochemical substances. One more benefit from nuts is that when combining them with greens oil will increase phytochemical absorption of fat-soluble chemicals that are in already healthy vegetables. We do not have to go low fat and avoid nut and seed consumption and predominantly eat starch. We should eat starch and nuts and all other food in wide variety possible. So far the science has not correlated high seed and nut consumption with any disease including obesity, except in people who have allergies. Just the opposite. They are beneficial in almost any condition. Brazil nuts are full of selenium, and walnuts are protective against cancer, lignans in flaxseed are one of the most protective chemicals against breast cancer and are also full with omega three oils for brain function. Our ancestors had been eating raw nuts and seeds for a long time. They are our natural food as much as fruits or grains or young leaves or other green leafy vegetables. The healthy diet is the one we had evolved and have adapted at eating. That is it.

Taste has nothing to do with it. It is not the tastiest diet. In nature, there is scarcity, so taste exists as a reward not as common theme for every meal. That is the reason why the story is the same everywhere. The bigger the poverty, the lamer the food, the more natural it is because baseline human condition is poverty and hunger. That is the normal state. Yes, I know you will not feel the same way, but that is the case. For every animal in existence in nature, hunger is the normal state of being. Alternatively, a constant struggle for food would be more precise. For every animal that lives on this planet, food obsession is a daytime job. Most of the time during their lives animals spend on searching for food. There are no supermarkets and cans of ready to eat meals. It is the struggle. Moreover, that was a normal condition for humans even today. Well, at least the body physiology part. Our desire and pleasure-seeking behavior are what makes us sick. Evolution did not predict electricity and microchips and cars. We are maladapted to our habitat. We have underlined mechanisms that force us to act in an evolutionary protective manner such as overeating on food. The not so unique obstacle now is that there is no scarcity anymore. Also, even worse, we eat stuff like meat that is not congruent with our physiology. And what is worse we eat it every single meal. And what is even worse we are surrounded with all of the toxic chemicals we never had to deal with in the past, and we do not exercise and move anymore and do not have enough of sunlight and do not have normal relations to other species and other humans. We are technology dependent, atrophied and poisoned. We are dependent on our food to be supernormal stimuli and everything around us to be supernormal stimuli. Supernormal is the new normal. Everything has to be supernormal now to be normal. From video games to movies, to drugs to game addiction, to porn addiction, and sex and violence in every frame. Eating kale is not for us anymore. Eating fruit is not for us anymore. The fruit was ones upon a time the highest treat we could find in nature. Ultimate dessert. What is fruit today? The hybrid derived from selective breeding to be sweeter. Had we ever in our life tried real wild fruit without altered genes? Even that over hybridized variety is no match to pure refined sugar, so we are going to drink colored sugar water like Coke and sodas.

All we need is McDonald's senior vice president for marketing who under oath in the court of law described Coca-Cola as nutritious because it is providing water. And yes this happened, it is not a joke. We had forgotten who we are. What we are. Confusion is self-inflicted. If you have any question what is healthy, go to nature. Ask yourself is this something that Homo erectus might eat and do. If answer is no, then we should not eat it either. Evolution works in millions of years. Yes, there is calcium in milk and protein in pork and iron in beef, but there is also saturated fat and cholesterol and hormones and toxins. In our natural plant foods, there are substances that we need too but are lacking in animal products like antioxidants and other phytochemicals and fiber. Food is a package deal. All for the price of one. And no there is nothing terrible in the saturated fat or animal protein or cholesterol. Everything can be eaten. There are plants that eat animals, whales that feed on plankton. There is only bad food for us. We are not anatomical omnivores, and we will suffer from maladaptation. We have to seek the optimal diet that is congruent to our evolution in a broad sense. We have to understand not what is natural but what is natural for us. There is nothing evil in eating meat if that is your nature. In our case, it is not. There would be a maladaptation and price to be paid both in terms of physical money and health and the environmental cost at the end. People have a problem with this because the food is an addictive substance. And unlike any other addictive substance, we cannot get away from it. Alcoholics just might cut all of it, don't buy it and avoid it. We cannot avoid food. We have to eat every day so our addiction is not curable one. We might get away with some of the animal products in the range of a couple of percents. More than that will have an impact on our health. Reality is that people will always eat meat. People will always smoke or drink. How many clubs and bars have we visited in our life? However, what will happen if bunch drinking and clubbing became everyday practice? We can get away with drinking maybe once a month but getting drunk every day is not such a good idea. The same story is applied to meat and all animal products. If you eat meat, then treat it as such, as a toxic substance like alcohol or drugs that are giving you pleasure or satisfaction. So do it in moderation. Smoking weed every day, not a good idea. Eating meat every day, not a good idea. Drinking alcohol every day, not a good idea. Also, that is just the beginning.

A vegan diet is junk if we just cut out the meat from the diet. Refined sugar and oil are vegan. Many people who became vegan do it for moral or spiritual reasons. They do not do it for the right reason, and that is self-understanding and self-comprehension. They are just emotional, and they want to be better than other people. And that is good too. But unless we truly understand and do broad spectrum analysis of our own nature in a logical way nothing will come out of this. Some vegans eat whatever they like and then substitute with supplements and powders. There are "soy boys" that eat the same as before just substitute meat with soy. There are pure junk vegans that eat just junk. French fries and chips and a bunch of different variety of sugars and sodas. Moderation of animal products is not a healthy diet it is just the beginning of it. Go vegan?

No. Don't go vegan. Go whole food plant based organic nutritionally optimized diet. Veganism is just the beginning. The first step. And no, you do not have to be vegan. Not everything has to be kale either. We can get away with a small number of animal products. The problem can arise because we are so removed from our natural habitat that most of the stuff we do is unnatural. So you will eat meat ones a month. You will probably eat some ice cream or chocolate or something else here and there. Then you would go to that party you are waiting for and drink a lot and use drugs. You might get overstressed at the job and get just too much caffeine. You might not get enough sleep one or two nights. Maybe you have some prescribed drugs that have side-effects. You drink tap water and don't eat organic so here are some more toxins, and here are some more from the environment. To release some tension, you might smoke some weed. Here and there. You are on your phone all the time, and there is all of that radiation coming from Wi-Fi, and you had long distance flight last week with some cosmic rays on your name. You see now how things can multiply.

And when I say nutritionally optimized, it might sound too scientific, and it is a form of scientific approach. It is a simple step that we can do to see if our dietary habits are giving us all the nutrients we require. When you clean your diet and cut all the animal protein and junk and oil and sugar and salt and chemicals and toxins both from food and environment and optimize your diet both in terms of macro and micronutrients, then you can check if anything is missing. There are a lot of small programs for PC or Android where we can add all the food we ate during a day. We can check the charts of nutrient content to see if we had all of the recommended daily values of all minerals and vitamins and other micro or macronutrients. For example, we can check for the most common deficiencies like selenium, iodine, magnesium, potassium, vitamin e, fiber. Most of the non-essential minerals and other secondary plant metabolites do not have RDA because science is not at that level yet, but they are important as much as the rest of information we can find in these charts. I admit that this can be a hassle, but we must analyze our dietary habits to see if we have some deficiencies. It is individual and specific for every person. You might eat more grains, someone else might eat more nuts and seeds, someone else might eat more fruit, someone else might eat more other types of starches, and you might be missing something important. After some time, you can have insight into your food choices, and after a while, with practice, you would know even if you do not look at charts if you lack in some nutrient. In the time it would become a habit, and you would not think about it anymore. However, for beginners who eat what they like, it is a challenge, and it is psychologically not acceptable for them to think of food in such a manner. Food for most of the people is not energy that has to sustain them. It is satisfaction, an emotion and this scientific approach is just ruining their meal. What usually occurs is that you might see that you lack some nutrient like iodine for example. Then you can start to balance your diet by incorporating food items that are the most abundant in iodine. So you will add some seaweed for example. In time this approach can optimize your diet and then you can start to enhance it.

We have some 2000 calorie daily allowance sort of speaking, depending on our basal metabolic rate. It is a number we can spend if we do not want to overeat and became obese. We can see if we can cut out something really bad and substitute it with something really good and still have our 2000 calorie balance. At least that was my approach. I started to look for the ways to add more nutrient for the buck sort of speak. Meaning more nutrient dense diet and especially more nutrient variety in the diet with all of different pigments and phytochemicals and all I found to be beneficial in research. I started to analyze what are, for example, antioxidant-filled foods, what are anti-microbial foods, what are cancer-preventing foods, so I started to add different items and weird herbs from Asian markets and so on. There is a lot of research that I will try to cover in this book series, but I cannot cover everything. I made a hobby out of it and form of science. In my case it is a hobby. In someone else's case, it might be necessary work due to illness. This is work that if you do it will increase your own self-knowledge and health. You do not need to have nutritional expert beside you. You can do this by yourself. Mineral deficiencies are the most common and also low fiber and antioxidant intake for the average person. If you are learning and reading this book, it might be a good starting point because you will learn much of the knowledge that I had to learn from scratch. Alternatively, in the end, you might don't do a thing. Most of the people do not care. The big problem is that in the end, we might don't care what we do, but nature does not care that we do not care. For every action, there is an opposite reaction. We might don't see it right now, but nature is not an unbreakable entity. Universal law of existence says that there is no free meal. If we poison our land and water because we need more and more at the end we will, not someone else, we will eat that same poison when it comes back to us thru food chain. We had already destroyed our oceans. Everything including nature has braking point. Chronic diseases are just the symptom and just the first one if nothing changes. Human nature is not correlated well with all of our achievements in technology. It is hard for us to sustain ourselves independently from evolutional conditioning. In reality, we are just drug addicts that suffered millions of years of starvation and now finally; we have our payback time.

Toxic overload

"Only when the last tree has died, and the last river has been poisoned, and last fish had been caught will we realize we cannot eat money" – Indian proverb

Earth is a planet. The planet is not just a planet. It is a closed system. Imaginary lines in human-made up charts do not stop natural processes. Water evaporates, winds blow, rain drops, the river flows. In closed systems balance exists. Everything that is without balance crates cascading effects that at the end create new balance again. Animals who seek the food from habitat cannot overpopulate because the food is going to disappear. Predators who feed on prey cannot overpopulate because there is no prey. They are all codependent. We might think that tigers are great and robust, but tiger life depends on finding the pray. The pray have power over the tiger existence because tiger depends on it as much as the prey depends on the plants that it eats. If the environment shifts, the balance is disrupted.

Every time balance is disrupted something is going to die. That is what balance in nature actually means. The species which are most agile and adaptive will go on the others will not, so evolution goes forward. There were many imbalances or great extinctions on this planet so far. The last one created conditions for the rise of mammals. At this point, we are, or we think that we are above natural order. We had ascended to godhood with use of reason and technology, so we do not consider our actions as a relevant factor when calculating the impact on our habitat. We can create deep underground bases where we can even survive the nuclear holocaust. We can grow our food hydroponically with UV lamps. On a personal level, we do not consider ourselves part of nature. We are scared of nature because we are not able to survive by ourselves in the wild anymore. Nature is our enemy. We always want more of everything, and we are never going to be satisfied as a consequence of evolutionary conditioning. To want more in an evolutionary sense means to have more chances for survival.

Because now we do not have any natural predators to lower our numbers we are going for more and more as much as we can with no end in sight. All stories about the goodness of our hart and how we need to care about our planet are nonsense. Every single one of us just wants more. Bigger house, better car, house on the beach, better-looking woman and more delicious foods and everything we can get our hands on. We cannot control our evolutional conditioning, and we cannot control our behavior. We will destroy everything that is weaker including weaker humans too. We will use natural resources and turn them into commodities, and we will use every available resource because it is the race. Another human is our competition. Scientific advances mean economic progress, meaning more advanced weapon systems and "freedom" from other humans and nasty people who have different views on reality and what life should be or for that manner even don't. It does not matter. They are other humans, and that is never a good news.

Undeveloped countries must advance because they are under foreign commercial exploitation and slavery. They must use everything possible to free them self from poverty. Developed countries must wage war for resources against them and against each other. And all of this is just a normal part of nature. More food, more water, more energy, more land, more destruction, more artificial fertilizes, more farms, more oil used, more factories and of course more war. If you do not want war or you do not want to progress your competition will. In that case, you are going to lag in the race of survival, and then the war will find you when scarcity hits the markets, and you are not going to have any chances then. That is what happened to communities that were not in a constant war like the Roman Republic was and later Roman Empire and later Colonial powers of Europe. The peaceful lagged behind and went extinct or went into slavery. That is human nature. That is progress. There is no other way. That is how evolution works. There is nothing evil about it.

We have successfully eradicated the entire Neanderthal race and many other species as well and who cares about that? The way we are evolutionary conditioned to survive is not cute or pretty, and we consider ourselves now to be a developed civilization. But we still lack the understanding that we are going to have to pay the price. Toxins in the environment and a whole variety of human-made misbalances are not going to disappear magically in the thin air. Toxins accumulate. Biodiversity shrinks. Heavy metals, chemicals, radiation, mutated organisms all of it enters the food chain and return to us on the plate. And we have a double problem. We have diets that are not congruent with our physiology that just by themselves will create all kinds of problems and diseases and on top of that we have a toxic overload in different varieties and forms that comes from same food and environment as a consequence of unnatural and technology-based systems.

Our way of life is entirely different now then the one we had in our normal and natural habitat, and we have to pay the price. However, wait oceans are enormous. How can something that insignificant to the scale of our planet create any problem? When toxins get into the environment, they will end up in water. Then trough river systems eventually will end up in the ocean. They will get diluted, and there will be no problem. In the time they will dissipate. The short answer is no. It is correct that concentrations of all of our heavy industry pollutants and drugs and other chemicals are low when measured directly in ocean water, but there is a phenomenon called bioaccumulation. If the chemical is stable, it will end up in plankton, algae and other organisms. If there is substance in the environment, the organism will absorb it, and that is a process known as bioaccumulation. When we breathe if there is smoke in the air we will absorb it in the same manner as plankton or algae will absorb anything that is in the water. If a rate of absorption is faster than the rate and the ability of the organism for excretion, the substance will in time accumulate. A substance such as heavy metals for example or pesticides that remain unaffected in the environment and are stable for an extended period will get filtered by the organisms that live in that water. Because they have the tendency to be soluble in fat but not in water they accumulate in living organisms. Meaning they stick to the fat and other cells in the body and don't want to leave.

Therefore, all the poisons that are in oceans and that are humanmade and are heat resistant and chemically stable will bioaccumulate and reach a much higher concentration in organisms than in water. Organisms are like filters. They filter everything that exists in water good or bad. This is not good news for us. The situation would not be even so bad, but there is one more process called biomagnification. If we understand the food chain, accumulation of toxins gets hundreds of time worse as we move up. These fat-soluble toxins cannot be metabolized or broken down, and at the same time, they cannot be excreted thru kidneys by urine because fat and water do not mix. The only way for the organism to get rid of them is by enzymatic activity, and if an organism lacks enzymes to degrade them, they will accumulate in fatty tissues. Most if not all of these chemicals are new and human-made and organisms do not have a mechanism to detoxify them because in evolution they never had to, until now. So what happens is that when small fish get eaten by big fish, all of her toxins get passed into the bigger fish. Fats and all toxins in them will be digested in the gut and will be absorbed into the organism of the predator where they will be accumulated even more. Since at each level of the food chain there is some degree of energy that is lost, to compensate a predator will consume more significant number of prey, including all of their lipophilic toxic substances.

Concentration may be insignificant in oceans, but then water starts to get filtered by algae. Two main groups of substances biomagnify. Both are lipophilic and are not easily degraded. One of them are these new chemicals that are unknown to the immune systems of animals. Those substances are known as "persistent organic pollutants" or POP's. They are called persistent because they do not degrade in the environment. Regular sewage water when enters the river or the ocean has no impact on a large scale because it goes through natural process of degradation and disappears. Only artificial human created unnatural chemicals remain, the persistent ones.

Beside POP's there are metals. Metals are elements which means they are not living matter, so they are not biodegradable. Organisms that had thru evolution been exposed to high levels of some of these toxic metals that can be found naturally in the environment did in time develop defensive mechanisms to counter that exposure. The problem arises when there is an abrupt shift in an environment that are exposing these organisms in higher concentrations then what they are adapted to cope with. That will cause a buildup of these metals in the body that is unable to detoxify them and excrete them rapidly enough to prevent damage. Mercury, for instance, is only present in minuscule amounts in seawater. When algae absorb seawater, everything in it including mercury will stick and won't leave. Algae in some sense are acting like a seawater filtration system. Mercury will get absorbed by algae (generally as methylmercury). That filtering will start the process of bioaccumulation. Any species that will eat algae will also eat all the mercury in it. That will result in an ever-increasing concentration and buildup in the adipose tissue of successive trophic levels with the ever-increasing level of toxicity all the way up to larger fish. When we or any other predatory species eats those large fish, we will also consume all of the accumulated mercury. As bioaccumulation increases the concentration level in the predatory fish or birds will be much higher and in some cases severely toxic. For instance, herring contains mercury concentration at approximately 0.01 parts per million (ppm). Top predator like shark will have it at even higher than 1 ppm. How did mercury even end up in the seawater? Inorganic mercury is found in the ground, and it gets released by gold mining and primary production of non-ferrous metals. The more substantial contributor is fossil fuel burning. When coal or oil is burned it will be released into the atmosphere then it will be washed by rain. Thru river streams eventually it will end up in the ocean. Once in the ocean, it never leaves for eternity. It does not biodegrade.

We are being taught to think of poisons in a dose-dependent manner because that how modern medicine works. Something is poison, but it has low concentration so it is ok. Some side effects and so on. "The dose makes the poison" (Latin: "sola dosis facit venenum"). It is an adage intended to indicate a fundamental principle of toxicology. It is credited to Paracelsus, the alchemist, and father of modern medicine. Now, this is correct for some chemicals but not for all of them. Some toxins do damage, and I will argue most of them do damage in any exposure. This means that if we ingest even one molecule of a substance, it would cause damage. That damage would not be enough to kill us, but it will happen.

An excellent example of this is mercury. It is so toxic for our brain that it kills brain cells upon contact. Neurologic damage is most severe in utero. Mercury upon contact with neurons causes neuronal atrophy. When it enters the brain no matter in what concentration, even one atom of it, it will do severe damage. If exposure is significant, it will cause severe neuronal atrophy with no chance for recovery. Long-term studies have demonstrated that even minuscule prenatal exposure at very low concentrations can cause a detectable loss in the areas of memory, language and motor function. Children are so sensitive to it, so if affected, they may have hearing loss, visual loss, seizure disorders, developmental delay and long-term stigmata including motor impairment. For a pregnant woman, it is forbidden to eat tuna in any amount. Also, your brain and body can be exposed to toxic mercury through a number of other ways as well, from getting a flu shot to having a dental filling. To be reasonable here, one can of tuna have more mercury in it then 100 vaccines. Studies have found that people with amalgam dental fillings can have mercury vapor concentrations ten times higher than those in people without them. Fish consumption provides nutrients but also provides methyl-mercury. All fish, not just tuna, contain methylmercury (MeHg), some more some less. Because the toxic effect of mercury is most destructive during brain development, prenatal exposure is of the most significant concern. Mercury is cardiac toxin as well, not just the brain one. I will give an example here to put things into perspective.

In this study (Fish consumption, methylmercury, and child neurodevelopment. Curr Opin Pediatr. 2008 Apr;20(2):178-83) they analyzed connections of children susceptibility to mercury both from pregnancy exposure from mother and from fish consumption. Thimerosal from vaccines was looked into as well and dental amalgam impact on child neurodevelopment. Vaccines in the past used something called thimerisol, which is preservative containing mercury. To put this into perspective. Eating a single serving of tuna had the same mercury level as 100 (one hundred) thimerosal vaccines. Summary of the study was: "Exposure to mercury may harm child development. Interventions intended to reduce exposure to low levels of mercury in early life must, however, be carefully evaluated in consideration of the potential attendant harm from resultant behavior changes, such as reduced docosahexaenoic acid exposure from lower seafood intake, reduced uptake of childhood vaccinations and suboptimal dental care." Thimerosal has been taken out from most of the vaccines young children get in 2001, with the exception of the flu vaccine, which still contains small amounts. There was a big public concern and mistrust in vaccines and possibility of links with autism and other diseases. Because mercury is a neurotoxin, it is thought it is the underlying cause of connection between autism and vaccination. Today more children get autism even without mercury in vaccines and estimate is that this number will grow. This is big subject to analyze, and I will say that most of the vaccines are dangerous and unnatural just by themselves and can cause harm but they do save a lot of children's lives and at the end, it remains the question of trust in the companies that supply these vaccines.

If the government or big pharma want, now I say "if" the powers at high places wanted to use mandatory vaccination to create sterilization or autism or some other disease later in life or something else they absolutely 100 percent can. It would not be possible to detect it and if you do not have the trust in the system then don't take the vaccine. In one case The Kenya Catholic Doctors Association saw evidence of the sterilization. Six samples of tetanus vaccine from different places around Kenya were sent to be tested. The samples were not sent to laboratories in Kenya but to the independent laboratory in South Africa. All six of them, not one, not two but all six tested positive for the HCG antigen. The HCG antigen is only used in vaccines for sterilization of woman. There is no other medical application. These vaccines were given to a woman and young girls of childbearing age. HCG (human chorionic gonadotropin) have different biochemical functions in the body with the most important one being to trigger ovulation. Without HCG embryo cannot be implanted in the womb. HCG is used as a fertility treatment if a woman has a problem with conception. However, when you inject HCG via vaccine as an antigen, then it is a different story. Your body will create antibodies to it. From that point on, like in any other autoimmune disease, the antibodies will be present until the end of life itself. Those antibodies will attack HCG and will cause the woman's body to reject embryos, effectively permanently sterilizing her. In this study (Anti-fertility vaccines. Vaccine. 1989 Apr;7(2):97-101.) the beta-HCG- TT vaccine evoked the production of anti-HCG antibodies in 61 of 63 women tested.

Dr. Ngare, the spokesman for the Kenya Catholic Doctors Association, stated in a bulletin: "This proved right our worst fears; that this WHO campaign is not about eradicating neonatal tetanus but a well-coordinated effective population control mass sterilization exercise using a proven fertility regulating vaccine. This evidence was presented to the Ministry of Health before the third round of immunization but was ignored." Be aware of this for your children health. Depopulation of Africa and the world is a big dream of the elites that drag it ruts back in the eugenics. At that time there was no outbreak of tetanus in Kenya. Because of the local flood WHO perceived the threat of tetanus and decided to vaccinate local populations. WHO and UNICEF use local disasters to vaccinate as many people as they can. First in line for vaccinations are mainly children and young women. These vaccines are distributed for free and WHO also offer financial incentives for the Kenyan and other governments to participate in these programs. When UN funds are not enough for the purchase of annual vaccine fees, Bill and Melinda Gates Foundation steps in. Most of the vaccines are unnecessary at this point and even in the past as well due to the increase in sanitation. Most of the lives were saved by sanitization and washing hands and personal hygiene, not by the use of vaccines. However, if they are clean and tested for purity, and from the trustworthy supplier, they can be useful for some of the deadliest diseases.

Scientist in the study mentioned above about fish consumption, methylmercury, and child neurodevelopment also included a warning for consumption of Docosahexaenoic acid (DHA) in conclusion. Omega-3 or chemically Docosahexaenoic acid (DHA) is fatty acid that has a role as a structural component of the cerebral cortex primarily but also entire human brain, retina, and skin. Meaning if you cut out fish from the diet you need to find some other source of omega-3 fatty acids that are not from fish. They know that people believe in eating fish as a healthy habit because of healthy omega three acids so they must find another source. From where did the fish get omega 3s in the first place I wonder? Supplements like fish oil are heavily polluted. America consumes more than 200,000 tons of fish oil a year. They concentrate the omega 3s but also concentrate all pollutants from fish, not just mercury but PCB's and insecticides and all others. The molecularly distilled is no different. It is just another scam. Molecular distillation of fish oil can only remove some of the toxins, but most remain. It has a fancy name, but so far it is useful only for lighter organic contaminants (Simultaneous quantitation of multiple classes of organohalogen compounds in fish oils with direct sample introduction comprehensive two-dimensional gas chromatography and time-of-flight mass spectrometry. J Agric Food Chem. 2009 Apr 8;57(7):2653-60).

The only possible solution for toxicity is to go lower on the food chain. Krill oil should be purer than fish oil. Krill have high mortality rate and live short and are low on the food chain so they would not have as many pollutants. Going all the way to sea vegetables is the best course without supplementation especially because we can get more other minerals like iodine and phytochemicals when eating sea vegetables in salad then just taking algae based or krill-based DHA supplement. Our oceans are by now so polluted that even low-level organisms can be contaminated. Especially after algae blooms and all of the neurotoxins that this form of algae can create. I used to like to eat squids on a regular basis. I considered them healthy because they have a low level of fat in them. I considered them to be the purest protein actually from all animals. I liked to compare them to egg whites. I was a regular protein kid from the gym. Squids have a high reproduction rate and should not be contaminated, except their inner organs actually are and the older the squid, the more cadmium can accumulate (Influence of Squid Liver Powder on Accumulation of Cadmium in Serum, Kidney and Liver of Mice Prev Nutr Food Sci. 2013 Mar; 18(1): 1–10). Cadmium poisoning cases something called Itai-Itai disease (itai-itai byo, "it hurts-it hurts disease") was the name given to the mass cadmium poisoning of Toyama Prefecture, Japan, starting around 1912. Cadmium is very toxic. The discovery of small amounts of cadmium in McDonald's "Shrek Forever After" drinking glasses resulted in fear and anger. This led to a nationwide recall over dangers that this toxic metal could affect young children. The biggest problem with cadmium is that it has a tendency to accumulate in the body. Our bodies have a hard time excreting it so that is why it will accumulate and generate toxicity and carcinogenic effects. Therefore, even small amounts in long periods can create many problems. The biological half-life of cadmium is 16 years. That means that half of the cadmium ingested will leave the body after 16 years. Even if the levels of the toxin in the environment are low and minute amount of toxic substance if ingested, because of the long half-life, there will be a risk of poisoning if exposure continues for an extended period of time. The longer the half-life, the higher the risk. In top vertebrate predators, cadmium levels can be very high in sub-polar areas remote from industrial sites (e.g., Faeroe Islands, Gough Islands, Kerguelen Islands). In contrast, in the shelf waters of industrial countries, top predators display cadmium concentrations that are lower than those in similar species from sub-polar areas. Diet contribution obtained from consuming cephalopods can explain this natural accumulation of cadmium. They eat squids whole, but we can cut them up and eat only meat without their livers.

What about fish? Who eats just squids? Cigarette smoke and seafood consumption today represent some of the dominant cadmium pathways of ingestion. However, the logical conclusion from all of this is that even the creatures on the lower levels of the food chain that have a high level of reproduction can in short period accumulate heavy metals and a whole variety of other toxins that we do not know about. Squid meet might be clean for now if we cut out the inner organs and chuck them out but what about all the other stuff that I did not researched. Is it possible to research every aspect of food that we consume? I can only go logically and cannot do nutrition research for every single thing. I used cadmium and mercury here just as an example. Good old led poisoning plus entire periodic table can be added to the list, and so far this is just metals. The wide variety of other chemical pollutants are also the concern. Even polar bears now have renal lesions, reduced bone mineral density, fatty liver, and chronic inflammation due to the food poisoning (Do Organohalogen Contaminants Contribute to Histopathology in Liver from East Greenland Polar Bears (Ursus maritimus)? Environ Health Perspect. 2005 Nov; 113(11): 1569–1574.). The dolphins to (Anthropogenic and Natural Organohalogen Compounds in Blubber of Dolphins and Dugongs (Dugong dugon) from Northeastern Australia Arch. Environ. Contam. Toxicol. 41, 221–231 (2001)).

Organohalogen compounds are PCB congeners, DDT and metabolites, chlordane-related compounds, and so on. The effect of POP on human health and also to the environment as well are real and even if we think that it is something we can ignore the situation is not as such. The international community made the intention to restrict production at the Stockholm Convention on Persistent Organic Pollutants in 2001. However, the real story is that we cannot. They are an essential part of modern agriculture and different type of industries. Not everything can be recycled and purified. POP can evaporate too and enter into the atmosphere. Because they are resisting breakdown reactions in the air and are stable, they can travel long distances. Then they will fall and be re-deposited. This results in an accumulation of POP in areas far from where they have been used or emitted. They can reach as far as Antarctica and the Arctic Circle. We do not have a clean life anymore because there is no natural way to produce food organically for billions of people on the planet.

Some of the most known POP are for example Polychlorinated biphenyls (PCB's), and Dioxins and Dichlorodiphenyltrichloroethane (DDT). PCB's are used in plastics, as additives in paint, in electrical transformers, and capacitors, carbonless copy paper and as heat exchange fluids. So no plastic and electronics without them. PCB's are poisonous to fish at high dosages, and correlated with spawning failure at low doses. In humans, PCB's are associated with immune suppression and sterility, and most exposure comes from food. Today one in six couples have trouble in conceiving a baby. The number of couples attempting therapeutic methods due to the problem of natural conceiving has risen dramatically in post WW2 period. A number of 15% of couples that are sterile are more substantial than in the past for example 100 years ago. Sperm counts in the average male have fallen by almost half in the past 60 years. Fertility is lower with all men and woman, and as a result 1 in 6 couples are sterile. Many experts blame this fall on the increase in environmental chemicals which have weak estrogen effects, such as DDT and PCB. An increase in estrogen levels in the general water supply, due to use of the oral contraceptive pills, has also been implicated. There are many chemicals in this world of today. In this study (Role of environmental estrogens in the deterioration of male factor fertility. Fertile Steril. 2002 Dec;78(6):1187-94) they measured the correlation between sperm count and environmental estrogens. When they talk about environmental estrogens, they do not mean phytoestrogens made by plants but xenoestrogens, pesticides like PCP, DDT or BPA from plastic and so on. The most of them were found in fish. Urban fish eaters have the highest average PE and PCB levels. In infertile men, the total motile sperm counts are correlated with their xenoestrogen exposure. They also found substantial correlations between PCB levels and ejaculate volume, motility, vitality, and osmoregulatory capacity. Higher PCB's levels were associated with sperm damage ($p < 0.05$). Phthalates were also significantly higher in the infertile men with higher phthalate levels being correlated with sperm DNA damage. Both PCB and phthalate concentrations were correlated with a decrease in total mobile sperm counts as well. The conclusion was that PCB's and PE's (phthalate esters) might be influential in the deterioration of semen quality in the general population with particular attention being made as a contributing factor to infertility in men. Sperm count was something in the line of 10 (mean motile) live mobile count in millions for fish-eaters and above 80 for vegetarians. Around eight times the difference. If fish does not make you sterile by lowering sperm count, it will cause reduced testosterone and other pro estrogen diseases both in men and in a woman too like breast cancer, early menopause, endometriosis, and thyroid hormones problems. Many of the pesticides act similar and have endocrine disruption potential. For example, we know that hypospadias, a birth defect of the penis where opening is not at the tip but on the other side of the penis is caused by fungicide Vinclozolin (Endocrine disruptors and hypospadias: role of genistein and the fungicide Vinclozolin. Urology. 2007 Sep;70(3):618-210). Do you still think that eating wild caught salmon is health promoting?

Dioxin is an industrial pollutant of Agent Orange story. Dioxins are also created as a byproduct of high-temperature burning. They are emitted when hazardous waste, hospital waste, and municipal waste is burned. Also, conventional combustion creates them like automobile emissions, coal, wood, and peat. So are we going to stop to drive our cars? We did cut out lead from gasoline, but that is just lead. Dioxins are scientifically proven to be a human carcinogen and have been linked to enzyme and immune disorders as well. In laboratory studies, they were also associated with an increase in congenital disabilities and stillbirths. Adverse health effects may include reduced testosterone, early menopause, endometriosis, cardiovascular disease, altered immune responses, thyroid hormones irregularities, diabetes and metabolism alterations, skin, tooth and nail abnormalities. During pregnancy, exposure can result in altered thyroid, immune system, brain, and reproductive organ development. Animal food is the primary source of human exposure to dioxins. EPA started testing Americans for dioxin levels back in 1982. "Only" after three decades of delays in 2012, they released new guidelines that would set limits on the safe exposure of U.S. consumers. The response of the industry was to put political pressure in the White House. American Meat Institute, National Chicken Council and other industry groups pressured the politicians that they are lobbying that with these new guidelines their products: "Could arbitrarily be classified as unfit for consumption." They used word arbitrarily disregarding the fact that classification is based on scientifically determent dioxin levels found in different food products. In their minds warning consumers about the risk could: "Scare the crap out of people," and "Have a significant negative economic impact on all U.S. food producers." However, that is not the truth either. According to the FDA, over 95% of dioxin exposure is coming through dietary intake of animal fats, not all food. So it is just the meat industry.

A number of chemicals just grow and grow. Most of them are secret. We do not have research what they do, and nobody is talking. In the period from 2001, Stockholm Convention list has been expanded to include polycyclic aromatic hydrocarbons (PAH) or at least some of the most dangerous ones and also brominated flame retardants and some other compounds. Moreover, all of this is just what is tested. We need to understand that nobody will finance the research into the toxicity of different chemicals primarily in the long run because that is not what is going to increase the profits. Quite the opposite it will just make business more expensive. There is a lot of undeveloped countries that don't care about long-run destruction. Most of the impoverished nations are going to do anything just to survive, and that is breeding ground for corruption and companies love that.

Most of heavy industries dump their toxic waste in third world countries without regulation and give some money on a side to some corrupted politicians even to this day. Some of the waste is transported from western nations and dumped there also. There is a market for this. If you have something that is too expensive to get rid of in the US, transport it to the third world countries and dump. No regulations. Beside dumping, there is a one even worse trend. Companies that choose to invest in foreign countries and by this I mean forms of substantial greenfield investment tend to relocate to countries where they could have the lowest cost of manufacturing, and that means the lowest environmental standards or the weakest enforcement. The pollution heavens sort of speak. Only waste from industries that cannot be allocated is transported and dumped. Or I would just ask this, what happens at the individual personal level? How many regular people will dump their mercury electricity saving light bulb in the regular dumpster? Not just in the U.S. but all over the globe. That mercury from light bulbs will eventually be released in the environment. Alternatively, people are also dumping hazardous waste in town dumps to avoid paying the fees charged by waste transporters. Everyone does it, especially people with high credit debt. EPA began regulating hazardous waste in 1976. Toxic waste dumps that are holdovers from the era before 1976 are still here and pose a threat. Also, there is the practice of illegal dumping that has created a large number of waste sites.

On the industry level it is the same. One EPA rule that governs industrial sludge has proved to be very controversial. EPA allows sludge filled with heavy metals to be used as fertilizers on conventional food crops that were intended to be sold directly to the public in supermarkets. Environmental and some other consumer protection organizations referring to some of the studies that have been done on the topic claimed that substantial and dangerous levels of heavy metals are taken up by plants. When people eat these plants, it can pose a health hazard and could have an adverse effect particularly on children. So if this is behavior of "democratically" elected government of heavy regulated U.S. what happens in countries like Somalia then? Undeveloped countries do not have borders when toxic waste is in question because toxic rivers flow right into the international ocean waters. Toxic water is just a small part of what is acknowledged as toxic. A big chunk of regular waste is toxic too, and a big chunk of regular foods, drugs, cosmetics and other industry additives are toxic too but how much they do not want us to know. And to make a point for people who have a hard time dealing with truth and regurgitate all the time that there is EPA. My question is where was EPA when Agent Orange was used on people?

Even during World War 2, there were several chemical and biological weapons programs conducted by the USA and British governments that were designed to develop herbicidal weapons. As part of these efforts, several herbicides were discovered. After the WW2 British government was the first one to actively use these newly developed herbicides and defoliants to destroy vegetation with the goal of depriving local population of food crops. It was during Malayan Emergency (1948–1960) that Britain targeted food crops as part of a starvation campaign to create genocide of the local population and to force insurgents into submission or death. Big democracy is spreading human rights by destroying poor people crops and starving them to death. After the Malayan war ended in 1960, the US as a cradle of democracy considered that the British use of defoliants was a legal tactic of warfare. Tons of these herbicides that were dropped eventually will end up in the oceans. At that time Secretary of State Dean Rusk advised President John F. Kennedy that the British had created a precedent for warfare with herbicides. There is one interesting question here. How is it that US army was able to destroy rainforest in Vietnam 50 years ago by Agent Orange, but today it is somehow impossible to destroy poppy fields in Afghanistan visible from any satellite or drone in the NATO-occupied country? EPA is just marketing for regular people who need to feel protected.

No one will actually protect them. Still, you believe in law and order and EPA and stuff. OK, I will answer the question I asked before what happens in Somalia, so that we can see how the real world operates. The Ndrangheta, an Italian mafia-type criminal syndicate from Calabria (Italy), has been commissioned by big companies to do toxic and radioactive waste disposal since the 1980s. Radioactive and toxic waste was loaded on ships, and then these ships were sunk off the Italian coast. In addition, radioactive and toxic waste cargoes were sent to Somalia and other developing countries. Ships were either sunk there, or radioactive cargoes were unloaded and buried on land. Legambiente, an Italian environment protection NGO, provided the public prosecutor's office with the evidence collected since 1994 regarding the disappearance of at least 40 ships in Mediterranean waters. And that is just what was found. The investigation took more than two decades and was still incomplete because no one in the Italian government, in reality, wanted it to go to the fullest extent and investigate people behind the scenes. They just blamed the mafia for it. In that period, Italian prosecutors have looked into more than 30 suspicious deep-water sinking's. The practice was to sink the entire ship full of toxic barrels right into the ocean floor. Investigators suspected (but were not allowed to investigate) that Italian and foreign industrialists have commissioned the Ndrangheta, and possibly colluded with government agencies as well, to use the Mediterranean as a dumping ground. In EU cradle of democracy and human rights, nuclear waste is dumped with military and governmental approval in the middle of the Mediterranean Sea. Italian mafia is just low level. Errand boys. When this story leaked out by one man Francesco Fonti, a former member of Ndrangheta speaking out, the "business" was moved to Somalia and other places. According to Fonti, a manager of ENEA (Italian National Agency for New Technologies, Energy and Sustainable Economic Development) paid the mafia to dispose of more than 600 drums of radioactive, toxic and who knows what kind of waste from US, Switzerland, Italy, Germany, and France. Waste was buried in Somalia after buying off local politicians. It is suspected that former ENEA employees in collusion with big western industries paid criminals to dispose of the waste in the 1980s and 1990s. Shipments to Somalia continued into the 1990s, while the Ndrangheta mafia clan also detonated shiploads full of toxic waste, including radioactive waste from hospitals, sinking them to the seabed off the Calabrian coast. Let's write this again. Waste from US, Switzerland, Italy, Germany, and France from unknown companies. I know who these companies are, but I cannot prove anything so I cannot name them. However, you know them also very well. Fonti personally sank three ships. He identified one wreck that he sank himself in 1992 loaded with 120 barrels of radioactive and toxic waste. It was recognized later by environmental workers as MV Cunsky. It was located 28 kilometers off the coast of Cetraro, in Calabria.

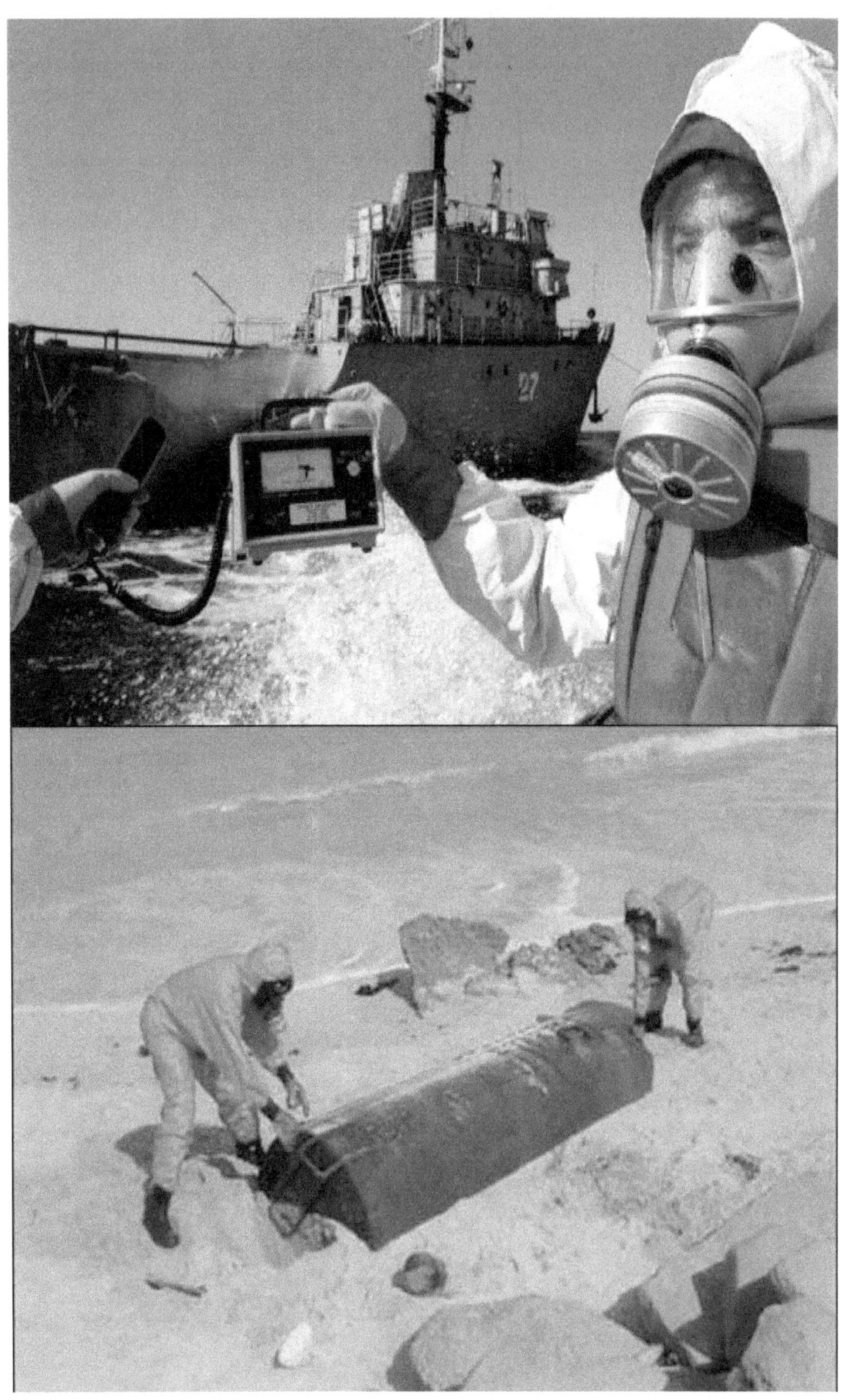

This is waste from western companies and industries that cannot be allocated to third world countries, so there is a need for disposal. For example, hospital waste fits the category. The same companies that research drugs and "cure" people from cancer and other diseases are dumping their radioactive waste to the Mediterranean Sea. Now take a pause in reading and contemplate on the level of corruption showed here. It involves shareholders of the top industries or western elite if you like. Most of them are not just into big pharma but banking and other important stuff. Basically, people at the top of all that you can think off colluding with international organizations, colluding with local "democratic" European governments, colluding with mafia stile syndicates, colluding with Somalia and other third world corrupt governments and controlling mass media like BBC, CNN not to report on these stories when they broke out. The same companies that have their government politicians talking about global warming and pushing that agenda for global taxation, i.e., carbon tax.

Now let me give another example. For people who do not know just background radiation had increased 600 percent from 0mSV in 1930, 1mSv in 1950 to over 6mSv today. As soon as radiation comes to "normal" values, agencies rise it to new "normal." According to Veterans Today, the average background radiation used to be 5 to 40 CPM, and now those readings are often above 1,000 CPM. In Japan, they raised the amount of radiation that even infants and children can be exposed to up to a maximum of 1 m/Sv per year to 20m/Sv per year, which is what full-time adult nuclear workers in the US are allowed as healthy adult males. There is also the concentration in the food chain of the radioactive materials too. And it is not just Chernobyl or Fukushima. It is all of that plus all of nuclear tests plus 3500 tons of uranium just dropped in Iraq war plus all other wars that we do not know what is dropped. And that is uranium (not depleted uranium) that US military got from all the old scraped nuclear bombs. What US military does is that they take enriched uranium warheads from old nukes and then melt them with the depleted uranium to make sort of mixture which is slightly enriched which is just about enough to make it legal. And other militaries do this too. Israel used enriched uranium in Lebanon and so on. Is this background radiation dangerous? I do not know. I will have to trust the institutions and say probably not.

However, it is not just the radiation. It is radiation plus, mercury, PCP, DDT, Dioxin plus entire list of forbidden chemicals, plus entire list of chemicals that are not forbidden but still are known to be toxic, plus on top of that all the bad habits from smoking to meat consumption full of dead bacteria endotoxins, plus prescribed drugs with side effects and list goes on. Different inputs are working to poison us. When we look at one of the poisons and say yes the concentration of that one is not enough to cause illness, but it will still cause some damage and damage multiplies in an extended time period causing diseases. Some of these toxins can work in synergy too. Organisms exposed to different types of POPs, can experience synergistic effects and have more overall toxicity then if they are just exposed to the same amount of just one particular POP (2+2=6 sort of speak). With synergistic effects, the toxicity of one compound is boosted by the presence of another compound in the mixture, and the end effects of combining them can far exceed the approximated mathematical additive effects of the compound mixture. Let us look at the history of most known of all pesticides the DDT. That will help us understand little better the whole picture.

DDT as all of POPs is stored in the fat of animals and takes many years to break down, and as predators consume the fat, the amounts of DDT biomagnifies. DDT is now a banned substance in many parts of the world, but it was not so once upon a time. DDT is tasteless, a colorless and almost odorless insecticide first discovered in 1874. In 1939 Swiss chemist Paul Hermann Müller discovered insecticidal action of DDT. That earned him Nobel Prize in Medicine. After the discovery with no long-term testing or anything similar the use of DDT skyrocketed. Immediately after the discovery it was pushed into use for WW2 military application to control typhus and malaria in troops but soon after it was used on civilians as well. By October 1945, DDT was available for public sale in the United States. It remained massively supported for an extended period by government and industry. A type of miracle substance. Diabolical weapon of modern science that kills billions of insects and saves millions of humans. The final solution to malaria and other insect-carrying diseases. Pesticides are neurotoxins for insects but not for humans. DDT in insects opens sodium ion channels in neurons, causing them to fire spontaneously, which leads to spasms and eventual death. All the bug needs to do is to walk over the treated surface. DDT is absorbed thru the feet and spreads to the entire nervous system. From 1945 to 1955 annual pesticide use went from 125 million pounds to over 600 million and even the suburbs were treated with DDT. It was considered absolutely safe and if people had problems with mosquitos the spray truck came and sprayed. They were told to stay inside for a few minutes until truck go by and that is it. Government endorsed the product, and chemical industry pushed it aggressively. In scientist's mind, it was just neurotoxin for insects.

They could not consider the likelihood that it might do other stuff in the long run. In the eyes of corporations and government when spraying it was logic that this product is cheap and effective so little is good but more is much better. Public Health Department staged demonstrations to convince the public of DDT effectiveness and safety. They sprayed it directly on children for demonstration. Example including public pools and school lunch areas where children were eating DDT enriched sandwiches. Planes sprayed over houses, whether people like it or not. In 1957 Massachusetts bird sanctuary was sprayed. It was owned by Olga Hawking's friend of Rachel Carson. The birds showed all the symptoms of DDT poisoning.

Carson later wrote the book named Silent Spring. It was published in 1962 and became a bestseller. In the book, she argued that the effect of massive DDT spraying is dangerous. At that time there were no long-term exposure research or data on what DDT might do to the human body. She warned that progress has a price. It was the seed of doubt in the minds of the people that completely believed the government in cold war era. She argued that: "These sprayed dust and aerosols are now applied universally to farms gardens forests and homes. Non-selective chemicals that have the power to kill every insect, the good and the bad, to still the song of birds and leaping of fish in streams. All this for the intended target may be only a few weed or insects. Can anyone believe it is possible to lay down such barrage of poisons on the surface of the Earth without making it unfit for all life?" Chemical industry and government responded with something in the line of: "The major claims in Miss Rachel Carson's book Silent Spring are gross distortions of the facts completely unsupported by scientific experimental evidence and general practical experience in the field. If man were to follow the teachings of Miss Carson faithfully, we would return to the dark ages, and the insects and diseases and vermin would once again inherit the Earth." It became a political issue, and Kennedy was pressured to force Public Health Service to "look into this." At that time government agencies assured the public that there is no short or long-term damage to humans exposed to low level of pesticides. The effect to the wildlife was ignored too because 3 to 5-year studies on rats did not show anything. Government agencies at the time did know that pesticide accumulates in the fat of humans, but that was not a big deal too because if accumulation does not reach levels that are necessary to be harmful exposure is not a problem. Public Health Service was ensuring people that there is no evidence that small doses of pesticides we get are causing harm. And there was no evidence because investigation actually at that time never had been made. The government was still assuring people everything is ok. In Silent Spring, Miss Carson was stressing the possibility that pesticide chemicals may be working long-range harm in man in ways, not yet detected perhaps contributing to diseases like cancer and leukemia and genetic damage. In the absence of proof, the government assured the public that everything is ok and that Miss. Carson is fearmongering and that these disease correlations are a possibility but not probability and that Miss. Carson is just spreading alarmism. In 1972, after more than 9,000 pages of federal testimony the head of the nearly founded Environmental Protection Agency, William Ruckelshaus, canceled DDT's registration in the U.S. However, it was a political decision. It did not answer the scientific question, does DDT cause a long-term environmental impact and does it have a long-term impact on human health as well? It was a political decision based on easing the public mind.

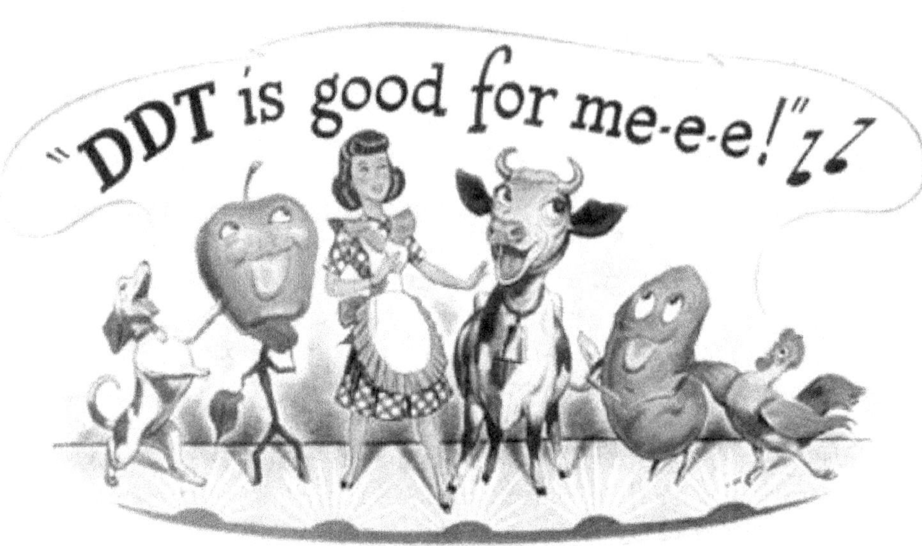

The great expectations held for DDT have been realized. During 1946, extensive scientific tests have shown that when properly used, DDT kills a host of destructive insect pests, and is a benefactor of all humanity.

Pennsalt produces DDT and its products in all standard forms and is now one of the country's largest producers of this amazing insecticide. Today everyone can enjoy added comfort, health and safety through the insect-killing powers of Pennsalt DDT products ... and DDT is only one of Pennsalt's many chemical products which benefit industry, farm and home.

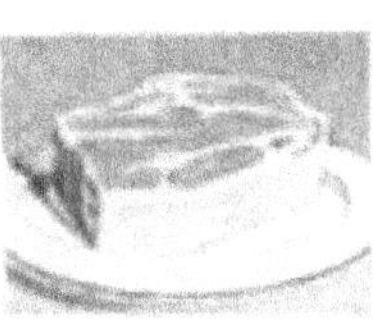

GOOD FOR FRUITS

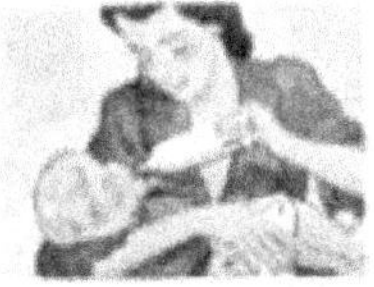

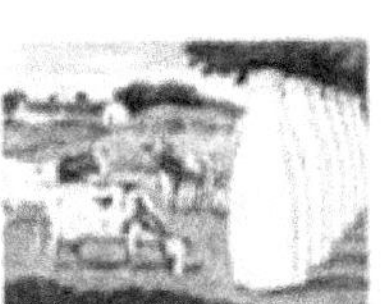

GOOD FOR STEERS

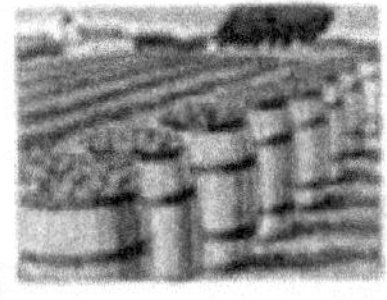

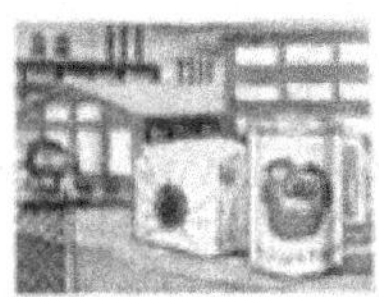

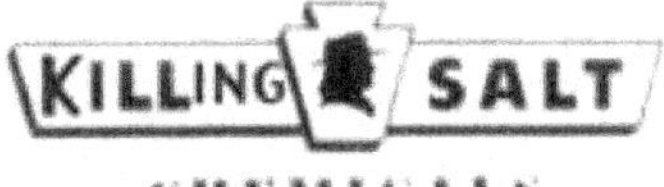

She longed for a Star Trek-type doctor with a state-of-the-art diagnostic tool. The doctor, with a few computer bleeps, would locate the exact cause of her newly discovered and doctor-baffling skin lesions and assign a painless treatment with no side effects.

We now know that pregnant women exposed to DDT have a significantly increased risk of premature birth. They are also at risk if they go full-term to have low birth weight babies. Studies in mice have found that DDE (DDT metabolite) blocks the binding of the hormone progesterone to its receptors. Home abortion pills like Misoprostol work by the same mechanism by blocking the binding of progesterone. It is the same mechanism of action with no difference. In the environment, DDT in some species that are more sensitive to it can cause extinction of entire species. For instance, DDT is linked with severe declines in bald eagle populations due to its effect on the thinning of eggshells. After DDT ban was in place, it took decades but bald eagle's numbers had returned to optimal levels, and they are not endangered species anymore. Because of its toxic effects, DDT is banned in the developed world, but in Africa, it is still used. It is cheap and can combat malaria which is two conditions that force the use of DDT to this day. It is understandable logic because if you are dying from malaria environment protection is not on your list of priorities. Different groups repeatedly attacked Carson. Africa Fighting Malaria for example and The Competitive Enterprise Institute blame the Carson for millions of deaths in Africa that could have been prevented with DDT. There is another problem in South Africa and also in some other countries as well. Malaria-carrying mosquitoes have developed resistance to the more expensive insecticide that has been used as a substitute of DDT named Pyrethroid.

So far studies have linked DDT and its metabolite, DDE to miscarriages and low birth weight, developmental delay, male infertility, breast, and other cancers, nervous system, and liver damage and cascading effect on the full range of different species in nature. However, to be clear, all pesticides are similar. Some are more toxic some less but all of them are toxic. There is not one single pesticide today that is health promoting. DDT just had to go because of the book and because people need to feel safe to buy products. A big chunk of pesticides used today are much worse than DDT. One more of the reason DDT was banned is that for 30 years it was overused and insects became resistant to it. It happens in an environment when poison is introduced.

Some bugs survive and multiply. Genetic characteristics of survivors will be more adapted against the same kind of pesticides. The pesticide used for the first time will have the most significant impact and will do more harm. However, some insects that survive will carry their genes forward. With time, forthcoming generations will be capable of withstanding its effects more and eventually becoming tolerant. Like mosquitos in South Africa. The longer time chemical is used, the more resistant insects became. It is the same story as antibiotic-resistant strains of bacteria. When this happens, the more effective and more potent and toxic poisons have to be used by farmers. That will repeat the cycle. New compounds are usually more expensive, so the economic cost will become higher and are also increasingly toxic. That generates a higher level of pollution and thus deteriorate the overall balance of the ecosystem even more. The high rate of reproduction of insects means that in a couple of decades they can become tolerant but what about you. Pesticides will run off to ground waters and streams and rivers. That will affect the biology of many species of fish, birds, mammals and other animals in a food chain eventually ending up in your body as well. GMO organisms are primarily created because of this so that pesticides like Roundup can be used in high dosages to kill all of this new resistant and nasty insects. We have reached the point where we have to alter genes artificially to keep the pace with natural evolution.

One good example is McDonald French fries. In every McDonald restaurant in the world, the fries are made from the same potato named Russet Burbak. This is potato from America that's unusually long, and it is also very difficult to grow. It has to be long because we like those red boxes with a little bouquet of very long fries visually. So McDonald insists that all potato be Russet Burbak. They also insist that all chips be clear without blemishes. There is one common defect of Russet Burbak called net necrosis. Because we like fries to be clean without brown spots on them, McDonald's won't buy potatoes from farmers who had them. The only way to eliminate the blemishes is to eliminate the aphids. The only pesticide that can kill them is called Monitor. It is so toxic that farmers who grow these potatoes have to spray the pesticides and would not go back to the fields for five days after the spraying. They have to wait for pesticides to wash off before they can go back. When they harvest the potatoes, they have to put them in atmosphere controlled sheds. In some cases, the size of sheds can rival football stadiums. The reason they are put into sheds in the first place is that they are not edible for six weeks. The potato has to off-gas all the chemicals in them.

The crop rotation is useful for addressing many problems of the over usage of pesticides. Monoculture excessively depletes the soil of certain nutrients. The rotation has a purpose of rebuilding the soil. One crop that leaches the soil of one kind of nutrient is then in the next growing season replaced by another crop that doesn't leach that specific nutrient but draws a different ratio of nutrients. In some cases, if done correctly crop rotation can even return that nutrient to the ground. Rotation in time will build biomass and fertility and structure of the soil from various root structures. When one species is grown continuously, year after year, it will in time build up the number of pests, and by rotation, the buildup of pathogens and pests will be mitigated. However, as a number of the human population has grown, monoculture with synthetic fertilizers is the only economically effective way to produce all of the crops we need. It is also left crops to be vulnerable to extensive attack by pests. Today we annually use more than 5 billion pounds of pesticides across the Earth and have altered genetics of many species creating superbugs. Colorado potato beetle, for example, is resistant to more than 50 insecticides. Other bugs get caught in the crossfire.

For example, since the late 1990s, there is an unexplained and sudden reduction in the number of bees. On the global scale, there are unusually high rates of decline in honeybee colonies. More than one-third of world crop production depends on bee pollination. The loss of biodiversity can explain it.

Due to monocultures that bees cannot use for food and the wide-spread use of pesticides, some of them can kill them directly or indirectly, the situation is now terrible. Bees dying reflects the dysfunctional balance in nature with a dysfunctional food system and flowerless landscape. In some sections of the world, there are no bees at all. In such places, people are paid to do pollination by hand. In the US, bees have been in decline since World War 2. There was around 4.5 million bee hives before the war and now the number is around 2 million hives. Food deserts are large-scale monocultures that do not provide any food to the insects including bees. The farms that use to support the life of bees are now food deserts dominated by one or two species like corn or soy with no flowering plants that bees need for survival. For example, the scale of almond monoculture is such that today 1.5 million hives or almost all of the hives in existence in the US is needed to do successful pollination. Hives are required to be transported across the US to pollinate just this one crop. They are trucked in in semi loads, and after bloom almonds are flowerless landscape with no food for bees, so they are needed to be transported to some other place to do pollination. The problem is that food production that requires bee pollination is rising annually. And then pesticides are necessary because monocultures are a feast for the pest that feeds on them. In pollen that bees collect there are at least six types of insecticides. There is one insecticide that is especially toxic for bees called neonicotinoid. Pesticides had improved over time and became stronger and more targeted, but still, they are not natural and still pollute soil, water, wildlife and our health too. Without them, food prices will skyrocket, and a big chunk of the human population will die from starvation or mosquito borne diseases.

Agricultural revolution had led to the rise of human population, and that is not something that can change no matter how much we encourage environment-friendly solutions. One thing, and maybe the only thing we are able to do is to lower our exposure by going organic and going low on a food chain as much as possible. Most of the pesticides and metals we get, we get from meat. There is a misconception that when we clean or wash pesticides from plants we lower our exposure. Most of the pesticide deposits cannot be removed by washing. They are mostly made on oily base so that rain won't wash them off. Correct numbers are just couple of percent overall. Washing the apple removes around 15%, and peeling removes around 85% but also removes most of the nutrition in the peal. If you do not eat organic and most of us do not, then do wash and scrub all produce thoroughly under running water. When you soak, there is no abrasive effect that running water provide. Running water will help remove bacteria (some of them may come from animal feces and be dangerous). There are also toxic chemicals on the surface of fruits and vegetables and dirt from crevices.

However, the real truth is that more than 80 percent of all pesticide exposure in the standard American diet comes from animal products, not from fruits or vegetables. I do not mean just fish with DDT and mercury accumulation from the ocean. Regular animal fat on farms accumulates toxins in the same manner.

Cows, pigs, sheep, and chickens are held in unsanitary and overcrowded conditions that exists on factory farms. To prevent pest infestation, they are directly sprayed with pesticides. Also, they are exposed to a large number of crop pesticides through their food. Animal feed sprayed with pesticides represent the primary source of exposure. Somehow we forget that all or most of the food that goes to animal feed are sprayed too. This is somehow not angulated by most people. By the estimates of the Environmental Working Group, every year in the U.S. around 167 million pounds of pesticides are just used to grow animal feed. These pesticides are eaten, and then they accumulate in animals. This can be allowed because there is no restriction in legal terms for pesticides used in animal feed. For instance, the most commonly used pesticide in the world is glyphosate. Legally, residues that are allowed in animal feed are more than 100 times then what is allowed on grains consumed directly by humans. Amount of glyphosate allowed in red meat that you buy in the store is more than 20 times that for most plant crops. These regulations have nothing to do with preserving public health, and nobody likes to talk about this because you cannot rinse pesticides out of meat, so this information is kept out of the public.

All of that poison is not going to disappear when we grill our burger magically. Most of the pesticides we eat or let say most of the people eat come from animal products. Meat cannot be peeled or washed. For farmed fish or seafood the same equation applies. Because of the increasing need for seafood and fish and the fact that our entire ocean is becoming depleted fish will mostly if not completely be farm raised as a rule. Currently over half of all fish is farmed. World Bank estimates that by 2030 around two-thirds of all seafood would be farm raised. The most common farm-raised fish are tilapia, salmon, catfish, sea bass and cod. Farmed fish have up to ten times more pollutants. Samples of farmed salmon have shown that it contains eight times levels of PCB's compared to wild salmon, four times levels of commercial beef and 3.5 times than other seafood. In couple of studies, they have analyzed more than 700 salmon samples from around the world. Most of these toxins are stored in the fat of the fish. It is the same story if we would compare game meat with the meat of farm raised animal. Much of the pollutants came from food that is given to the farmed fish. Food is the same as food for other farm animals and if chicken and pork have bioaccumulation of POP's so would the fish but because the fish are enclosed in water tanks the situation get worse because fish then starts to accumulate the pollutants from water as well. Fish waste and also uneaten feed will drop to the bottom beneath these farms and start to decompose. Average size salmon farm will produce the amount of excrement equivalent to the sewage of a city of ten thousand people. It is the breeding ground for bacteria that consume oxygen, and oxygen is vital for marine animals especially for shellfish and other bottom-dwelling sea creatures. Also, the excrement of the animals themselves is used as a fish feed. Chickens only use up to 30 percent of the nutrients from its feed. That means that 70 percent of nutrients is still in its droppings. Fish can eat those droppings and absorb all of the remaining protein, carbohydrate, vitamins, and minerals. These droppings if uneaten will also fall and settle at the bottom. Then, with time, insect larvae will develop, and the fish will eat the larvae that are filled with pollutants from the excrement themselves. Not only that but the transfer of pig waste is common practice too. It is an economically sound design technique known as integrated livestock-fish farming. Waste from chickens, ducks, and pigs are transferred directly to the fish farms. Fish like tilapia and carp use plankton as a primary food source. If the dosage is right, manure will give a massive boost to growth to the plankton in the pounds. This fertilization of the fish pounds will dramatically improve the fish growth and the level of toxicity.

Because in farms fish do not eat wild food only the feed they lack astaxanthin. Astaxanthin is red pigment from algae that algae use as a defense against UV light and represent one of the most potent antioxidants in marine habitats. The pink color of salmon and for example, the pink color of pink flamingos are a consequence of astaxanthin consumption. Pink flamingos are born white. In farming conditions, fish lack a wide variety of phytochemicals that they will naturally eat in the ocean, so they are given dyes. Farmed salmon regularly has dye added to it. Die is synthetically produced carotenoid astaxanthin that is used as a colorant. It even has different shades that range from carophyll pink from Roche to lucantin pink from BASF. These dyes are a scam. They have no purpose. Their only job is to fool you, the consumer, into thinking the product is natural looking, healthy and flavorful. Beside farming waste, the crowded conditions that these fish are in will lead them to be more susceptible to disease as well. It can be compared to regular farming which is breeding ground to infections and parasites. In ocean fish is scattered and infections will typically exist at the minimal level. In densely packed oceanic feedlots, diseases and parasites can run rampant. In order to cope with these conditions farmed fish are vaccinated as minnows. After vaccination fish is always on antibiotics and pesticides. One of the most significant problems for the industry is sea lice. In the wild usually, it is not problematic at all, but in the fish tanks, it is an entirely different story. At the first sign of an outbreak, farmers will add substantial amounts of pesticides to the feed. Because they are fed with fish feed, they also lack omega three fatty acids. Fish in wild get omega three from algae. Fish feed is nothing more than grounded fishmeal and vegetable protein and that mixed together with the help of binding agents such as wheat. In all types of fish examined, the amount of omega three fats was considerably higher in wild fish. Generally, farm-raised fish will be cheaper, will have 10-30% more fat than wild-caught fish (and that is not omega-3 fatty acids as a propaganda regurgitate but just fat which you already get too much of) with a higher level of toxicity and lower level if any at all of omega three acids. The solutions are closed systems. They treat and then recycle water and don't contaminate nearby wild habitats but that way of fish production is much more expensive, and we forgot that wild fish is polluted just by itself. Inflammatory potential of clean, unpolluted fish just by itself is far higher than that of a hamburger or pork bacon. Also, then we have pollution on top of that. If you think that eating salmon is healthy, you as well might just go with the bacon. All farmed raised fish and shrimp are just a poison. Shrimp and tilapia are the one of the dirtiest. Most of the shrimp and tilapia that you see in the markets and stores are from farms.

There is something also called cannibalistic feed biomagnification. Mercury is not just in fish. We feed a fish meal to other farm animals. Even to the cattle. Farmers discovered that if they feed animal protein to the cattle by mixing it with other plant food sources, cattle tend to grow more and produce more milk. It is not just humans that can eat animal protein all plant eaters can eat animal protein if the protein is first heated and treated even grazers. Psychologically we think we are omnivores because we can eat thermally processed meat but that is not the case. If you do not believe me here is one study (Effects of feeding a fish meal to cows on digestibility, milk production, and milk composition. J Dairy Sci. 1992 Feb;75(2):502-7). In this study conclusion was that: "There seems to be a good reason to feed a good quality protein like a fish meal to cows producing more than 30 kg/d of milk." Fish-eating cow's produce a milk that has no aftertaste, so yes this study was a success. Except for mercury. We get saturated fat from milk and meat and all of the rest of bad stuff, and as surplus, we also get mercury from fish in the milk of the cows too.

When we test all of the food products for toxic pollution levels, the number one is fish number two is chicken. The two "healthy" types of meat. Cheese comes the third. Worst then butter or bacon. We also feed all of the slaughterhouse waste products of animals to other animals. Because of the cannibalism the pollutants just circle around. The economically well-designed but extremely toxic trend among affluent countries is to feed any animal byproducts that cannot be eaten by humans to poultry and ruminants (herbivores such as sheep, cows, and goats). In industry, nothing is wasted including bones, manure, blood, heads and so on. Most of it goes to dog food or animal food. All of the blood, bones, and even roadkill corpses, supermarket waste meat, anything from the city shelter, work animals, euthanized pets and any protein no matter how decaying are grounded together, then heated to sterilize them, then dried and then used as animal feed. It is all part of rendering business. Inedible dead-animals and that means all of them including dogs and cats and other dead pets like reptiles, insects, or anything that is no longer alive, end up in feed used to fatten up future generations of their own kind. Protein is a protein. What cannot be used as animal feed or in other words that can be extracted for more expensive products will end up transmogrified into rubber, car wax, paint, and industrial lubricants. Some of it even goes to animal feed for chicken or fish and will not be used for pallets for pets meaning it will end up eventually in our own kitchen table. Most of the toxins that are thermostable will persist from one species to another. Prion disease is one good example what can come out of this (Mad cow disease). Not only are harmful prions found in the meats of animals, all other pollutants just get passed from one animal to another and eventually will end up on our own plate.

The logical step is to minimize the exposure. One of the ways is going low on a food chain, and other is eating organic. The only thing we can do. Go natural. Natural meaning natural human diet. Diet low on the food chain. If not, we will get exposed to neurotoxic substances like mercury and lead and endocrine disruptive substances like POP's and all of the carcinogens and pro-inflammatory compounds with systematic and chronic effects on our health. There are even levels of prescribed drugs in wild fish. Most of the drugs we take are extracted in urine and can end up in waterways. Drugs that are stable like Prozac, for example, end up polluting waterways. Chemicals we do not drink but use for cosmetics like hair dyes or creams with hundreds of different chemicals like paraben for example also end up in waterways. Several studies had confirmed the presence of trace concentrations of PPCPs (Pharmaceuticals and Personal Care Products) in all types of waters. Surface water and finished drinking water has it. Do they pose any health risk is largely unknown. The concentrations are low, but there is concern that some of them can bioaccumulate. The point of this argument is that even the small pills that people take time to time like ibuprofen can be detected in the environment. Dumping the tens of thousands of tons of chemicals produced in factories every year that do not degrade and stay in the environment for eternity, usually is not a got thing. If we count all of the industries around 700 new chemicals are introduced into the US market. That is just the US without any other country in the world. In the US alone more than 84,000 chemicals are used in processing, manufacturing and other types of industries. This does not count all the drugs from the pharmacy. These chemicals are everywhere, but the scary fact is that there is no safety data on most of them. They are in the water, air, soil, our food supply, and everyday products. Some groups of people also have higher exposure to these toxic environmental chemicals than others. For instance, workers who work on farms have higher exposures to chemicals used on the crops. Another especially susceptible group is a pregnant woman. Some pollutants can have a negative impact on fetus development. The amount of pollution in the environment will affect fetus much more than the mother. When they tested the U.S. pregnant woman in a study done in 2011, they found that almost all of the pregnant woman had toxicity from multiple chemicals and with some that were banned since the 1970s. Every couple of years CDC measures the number of environmental pollutants in bodies of Americans across the country. In this study (Environmental chemicals in pregnant women in the United States: NHANES 2003-2004. Environ Health Perspect. 2011 Jun; 119(6):878-85.) they analyzed biomonitoring data from the National Health and Nutritional Examination Survey (NHANES). Analyzing data for 163 chemicals they find that certain pesticides, toxic solvents, endocrine disruptors, carcinogens, and heavy metals were detected in 99–100% of pregnant women. On average pregnant woman is polluted with around 35 different chemicals including both banned and contemporary contaminants. Chemical cocktail levels of many of these chemicals were comparable to the levels incorporated in investigations and studies dealing with pregnancy and in levels that can have fetal adverse effects. Pregnant women were exposed to multiple chemical cocktails at one time, many of which can affect the same adverse outcomes later in life. Having one or two chemicals is bad enough but having 35 of them all the time and having hundreds of them running thru your body from time to time is toxic overload with synergistic effects that will have a significant impact on your health from reproduction to chronic inflammation to full-blown disease. If you want to become pregnant and decide to detoxify the short answer is that you cannot. Detoxification depends on the individual half-life of these pollutants with the presumption that you would never have any pollution in your life again. Which is not possible no matter what you do. In this study (Impact of adopting a vegan diet or an olestra supplementation on plasma organochlorine concentrations: results from two pilot studies. Br J Nutr. 2010 May;103(10):1433-41.) aim was to design the diet to prevent or reduce the body load of organochlorines (OC) in humans. Organochlorines are chemical compounds that were widely used after World War 2 as insecticides in the industry but were banned in the 1970s. They are resistant to degradation, so they still continue to be present in most of the food chains, and because they are fat soluble, they accumulate in the adipose tissue of organisms. Study 1 compared plasma OC concentrations between vegans and omnivores. Study 2 looked into dietary fat substitute olestra. They wanted to test if olestra could prevent the increase in OC concentrations that happen during dieting. What they observed was that OC plasma concentrations were significantly lower in vegans. In conclusion, there was a trend toward significantly lesser contamination in vegans than omnivores, and olestra did not prevent plasma hyper-concentration of the OC during ongoing weight loss. What surprised the researches is that vegans had as much as they did because theoretically they should not be exposed to a high degree to these pesticides. Vegans tend to have around 30 to 40 percent lower plasma concentrations. The conclusion was that vegans may be exposed by mother milk at the time of lactation and that becoming vegan or vegetarian is often a decision that is made in adulthood. Thus the omnivore diet during childhood and puberty result is contamination that is still detectable in adults. In addition, vegans may occasionally depart from their diet and eat animal products. Detoxification is a slow process and cannot be done on a weekend of detox diet cleansing or fasting. Detox starts with clean food. If we chose to go vegan, we would still get exposed because we live in our environment, not in a bubble. Most of the plant food has some of the pollutions in them. Some have more pesticides or heavy metals, or another type of toxins some have less and even organic food is not truly organic because it will pick up some of the toxins from the environment. We could not have clean food in the filthy environment only thing we could hope for is cleaner food, and that cleaner food is much more expensive, so if we look realistically, we will get exposed no matter what we do.

Realistic minimization of overall toxic load should be our goal. Every year Environmental Working Group releases the edition of the Shopper's Guide to

Pesticides in Produce, also known as the "Dirty Dozen." The guide is based on an analysis of the U.S. Department of Agriculture's Pesticide Data Program report. In the annual report from 2017 around 70 percent of 48 non-organic produce samples tested positive for at least one pesticide. Worst was strawberry samples with 20 different pesticide residues. There was also spinach, apples, celery, grapes, tomatoes. We should get familiar with this type of lists at annual bases because we might decide to go organic with some of the products or to avoid them or to peel them if possible. There is also a clean 15 list with might help us decide if we are going to buy products from this list more often or if we would by-products that are clean and regular instead of organic. The Clean 15 usually are sweet corn, and onions, cabbage, cauliflower, frozen sweet peas and a bunch of fruits we would peel anyway like avocados and pineapples. Other plant foods have a high level of pollution that are not sprayed like arsenic in rice for example. It happens naturally without direct human intervention. Arsenic is a typical element found naturally present in the soil, water, and air. It can also be the result of human activity such as mining or use of certain pesticides. Inorganic arsenic is listed as a class one carcinogen. The plant absorbs arsenic as it grows. Some plants will absorb more than others.

Rice absorbs the highest concentration among all commonly eaten foods. It contains between 10 to 20 times more arsenic for example than other cereal crops. Because rice grows in flooded conditions arsenic in the soil is released and more readily available. That released arsenic will be absorbed by the rice plant, and some of it will end up in rice grains. Because arsenic is already naturally found in the soil, it will be absorbed regardless of farming practices. If there is pollution of water even if the rice is grown organically the concentrations will be high. High exposures of people are reported in different areas of the world, especially in part of Asia and South America. China and Bangladesh have a problem with arsenic leaching to drinking water. In some part of China and Bangladesh drinking water is thoroughly contaminated with high levels of arsenic. From 2004, in the EU a stricter precautionary standard for maximum total arsenic of 10 μg/l in drinking water came into effect but to be fair EU never had a problem like China so for EU it is easy to adopt strict standards where there are no problems in the first place. Like any other poison, children are more exposed because they will typically consume more per unit of body weight as well as having more particular eating patterns and limited dietary choices. For instance, rice is used in many first foods. If we calculate dietary arsenic exposure in children per kilogram of body weight, it is estimated to be about on average 2- to 3-fold that of adults. High levels are found in most of the rice-based foods and drinks widely used for infants and young children. Low levels of arsenic impact fetus or children on different levels like growth development, immune development, they impact IQ development as well. In 2004 one study was done in Bangladesh that showed that children that were exposed to arsenic in drinking water had much-lowered scores on standardized tests. In 2013 one study showed that pregnant women who were exposed to even tiny amounts of arsenic in drinking water had children that had significantly more chance for developing respiratory problems. In Sweden, their National Food Agency (SNFA) have an official recommendation that children under the age of six do not consume rice in any form especially rice cakes. Rice cakes have more arsenic than any other rice product, and recommendation for an adult is also to cut down on consumption of rice cakes if they eat rice on regular bases. Children should have a balanced diet based on different grains as a source of carbohydrates and infants, and young children should avoid eating rice at all especially rice cakes and rice drinks. Prolonged exposure to arsenic in adults is associated with an increase in heart disease as well as lung, skin and bladder cancers.

There are steps to take if we want to eat rice to lover the arsenic content, but it will vary depending on the type of rice, the way it was processed, condition and place where it was grown and the way it was cooked. The highest concentration is in the bran. Rice bran should not be eaten at all so any product that was made out of it, for example, commercial rice milk would have higher concentrations. If we look geographically, the U.S. is the most polluted place. In modern poultry farms, there are too many of the chickens concentrated in the small amount of space. Most of them spend their entire life barely moving. In this type of conditions chicken manure is a problem for the creation of infectious disease outbreaks. The typical chicken will produce roughly 90 pounds of manure. In big farms, there can be hundreds of thousands of chickens in one facility. The floor of these buildings is covered with feces, soybean, ethers, peanut and rice hulls. To stop the infections and to prevent disease and to promote growth the poultry industry has used organoarsenicals, such as a 3-nitro-4-hydroxyphenylarsonic acid (Roxarsone, ROX). Roxarsone is just arsenic acid, and it is included in chicken food as anticoccidial and mainly excreted unchanged in feces. This arsenic added to poultry feed as Roxarsone ends up in poultry litter and then stops spreading of infections. Microorganisms will biodegrade and metabolize the Roxarsone into different toxic compounds one of them being arsenic.

Due to continued soil accumulation, soil arsenic concentrations from long-term poultry litter applications can exceed safety level standards. These compounds would leach and contaminate underground waters that are in some cases even used for human consumption. What is much worse is that chicken litter is used for application to agricultural lands and for fertilizing fish ponds. In the US around 90 percent of poultry litter filled with arsenic will be used in the agricultural fields as fertilizer. Then some of that arsenic will be absorbed by crops that grow on that arsenic amended field. Poultry litter has also been used as feed to the beef cattle as well. It is used as a starting material in the creation of mushroom compost. For years mushroom concentration of arsenic has rivaled the rice. The latest study showed that now mushrooms average around half of the rice. The estimate was that around half a million pounds of pure arsenic were dumped in the environment every year in U.S. FDA, monitors arsenic content in diets of Americans for decades. The highest concentration is in farmed raised fish 1.14 ppm. Fish are fed with chicken manure. Even if you avoid fish, lower concentrations were found in most of the food items analyzed. Chicken has 0.08 ppm and rice 0.16 ppm. Rice is the primary source of arsenic exposure in the non-seafood diet. FDA toxicologists argue that the average daily intake of arsenic poses no hazard to the consumer. I tend to disagree.

Arsenic pesticide usage in the U.S. has been common practice in cotton growing as well, so states like Mississippi and Arkansas have a higher level of pollution. Arsenic pesticides are now banned, but all of that pollution is still there so Californian rice, for example, have 41% lower level of arsenic then Mississippi one. The concentration of arsenic in the soil can be at the point where it affects the rice plant itself. There is an arsenic toxicity disorder in rice called straight head. The symptoms range from an increase of blank florets to complete grain failure. To deal whit this the industry created arsenic resistant strains. Now rice can take much more than previously naturally possible without getting any problem. The only thing left to deal with this situation is for the industry now to create arsenic resistant humans. The same story as with wine. Decades of arsenic pesticide use accumulated arsenic in the soil, so there is a constant, pervasive presence in American wine.

In this study (Cancer and non-cancer health effects from food contaminant exposures for children and adults in California: a risk assessment. Environ Health. 2012 Nov 9;11:83.) the California children were tested for exposure to multiple dietary contaminants. Cancer safety levels were exceeded by all children (100%) for arsenic, DDE, dieldrin, and dioxins. In past times it was rarely the situation where the entire population was poisoned, every single one participant measured with no exceptions. Also, safety non-cancer benchmark level for acrylamide was exceeded by 96 percent of preschool-age children, and also 10 percent of children were above safety levels for mercury. Acrylamide is substance recognized as a carcinogen by the U.S. government agencies. It is created in high temperatures in reaction with starch. So any fried and baked starch-rich food is filled with it like bread, French fries, potato chips, and cookies. What is important is the level of exposure. When FDA toxicologists say that they believe that the average daily intake of arsenic, pose no hazard to the consumer I say that I do not believe in their honesty. The one thing we can do is to apply logic, not belief. Believe in reason, not in government. Only scientific studies are a good reference for the truth, not belief into the system where corrupted industry officials are put into work in governmental institutions to give validity to their lies. The study showed that the real level of arsenic exposure was more than 100 times of acceptable daily levels for adults. More than 100 times the value not more than 100% in value. I want to write this again. More than 100 times of acceptable daily levels. For children and preschoolers, it was about 300 times. Let me write this again. 300 times more. "I want to believe" too, and I like the X-Files but not in FDA lying corrupted toxicologists. The ratios of excess expose in this study (how many times more above safety level the exposure level is) was as follows: 2–12 for DDE, 116–297 for arsenic, 18–

67 for dieldrin, 4–5 for chlordane (among children) and 202–1010 for PCDD/Fs. Yes, it is up to 1010 times the allowed values for Dioxin (PCDDs).

Figure 2

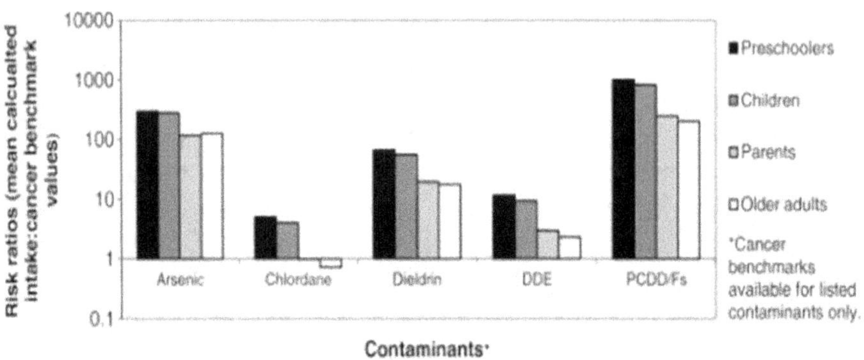

Hazard ratios of Cancer Benchmarks for contaminants.

Dieldrin was created as a safer alternative to DDT but was banned two years later in 1972. When we look into what food products are the most contaminated they were similar throughout all age groups. Meat, dairy, potatoes, and cucumber are most contaminated with POPs (DDE, dieldrin, chlordane, and PCDD/Fs). Until 1988 when chlordane was banned, it was used for home termite control and citrus crops and corn. Also, major POPs contributors were freshwater fish, poultry, mushrooms, cantaloupe, pizza (children only) and spinach (adults only). When we look at pesticides that are in current use (endosulfan, permethrin, and chlorpyrifos), the main contributors are celery, strawberries, grapes, tomatoes, apples, peaches, pears, peppers, spinach, broccoli, lettuce, and green beans if we don't count the levels in animal products. For arsenic exposure, farm-raised salmon, tuna, poultry, and mushrooms were top contributors in all age groups. For acrylamide exposure chips and all other types of fried potatoes like French fries, crackers, cereal for all age groups. For mercury exposure, it was fish and especially tuna. Dairy products are also the main contributor for chlorpyrifos exposure among children and lead exposure among all age groups. One of the top contributors was dairy and in some cases the main contributor of PCDD/Fs exposure, DDE and chlordane. PCDD/Fs exposure from dairy was more pronounced in children due to lower dairy (and higher meat) consumption in adults.

For ordinary people, it might come as a surprise that milk in addition to meat was found to be a significant source of pesticides. This is a consequence of the use of chlorpyrifos on grazing fields and feeds given to cattle. This practice is forbidden in organic milk production. Milk is one of the leading sources of POPs. Fish was a significant source of arsenic, dioxin, dieldrin, chlordane and DDT intake. Problem with chemicals like POPs is that they have the ability to accumulate in animal fat. So avoiding animal fat by decreasing consumption or choosing the lowest fat option of meat, dairy and fish is one strategy to lower the exposure. Another strategy to avoid the toxicity that will have better result will be to consume a plant-based diet. In the case of rice, some strategies can lower the exposure, but in essence, nothing can be done because it is a plant that naturally absorbs more arsenic from the water in which it is growing. The situation is just worsened dramatically in the US because of the use of arsenic pesticides, and now the soil is polluted. On 31 December 2015, the FDA withdrew approval for the last of the arsenic-containing drugs. It should be noted that EU has never approved the drugs containing arsenic for animal consumption. So as of 2011, due to the consumer pressure, the use of arsenic as feed to the chickens is banned in the US. Why this practice lasted so long and better question will be why use arsenic at all if we know the history of the substance.

The first mention of arsenic in history was at the court of the Roman Emperor Nero by Greek physician Dioscorides in the first century. Arsenic is a hazardous substance because it lacks color, taste or odor. It is abundant in nature and readily available to all classes of society. Because it can be mixed with drinks or food and leave no taste or smell it is an ideal substance for sinister uses. Symptoms of arsenic poisoning are also tough to detect because they mimic regular food poisoning and other common disorders. In a large dose, it causes vomiting, diarrhea, violent abdominal cramping, and death. With chronic poisoning in small doses, there would be confusion, loss of strength and paralysis. Eventually, arsenic trioxide (As_2O_3) known as white arsenic was commonly used to poison people with lethal dose the size of a pea. Pope Alexander VI and his son, Cesare were, for example, well-known arsenic poisoners. Pope, Alexander VI appointed cardinals and with privileges and power granted by the church, cardinals were encouraged to do whatever it takes to increase their personal wealth. Then at some point, they were invited to have a meal with the Borgias resulting in the death of the cardinal. In that scenario by church law ownership of cardinal property reverted back to the church or in other words to Pope, Alexander VI, his executioner. With its colorful and long history, arsenic is not a substance that people want in their food. In 2000 the biostatistics student came to the USDA in search of the project for his master's degree. What he was found is that arsenic level in chicken was three times as in the other meats. Although this was an unexpected finding, it was soon explained to him that in the USA antibiotics containing arsenic are fed to the poultry to promote growth, improve pigmentation and prevent diseases. FDA approved the first drug Roxarsone in 1944. So while arsenic-containing drugs were in wide-scale use since the 1940's the recognition of the exposure were only accrued after statistical analysis of the data. In other words, the FDA deliberately did nothing.

Student did his master publication. After that, study was published in 2004, expended in 2006. Again it was all the same story as before with Silent Spring. Only when consumers find out something and get angry the government (govern the men for the interest of elite) pretend that people interest are their concern. The National Chicken Council said that: "Contrary to assertions chicken production is not a major source of arsenic in the environment and that wide variety of food are contaminated with arsenic." Some of the chicken companies use animal health products that have organic arsenic-containing compounds in their makeup. Because the type of arsenic used is in organic form, not the toxic inorganic form made infamous in Arsenic and Old Lace the FDA approved these drugs as safe. This might seem logical to you, and I will like you to stop the reading and think about this. How is it possible that FDA approves drugs for 70 years that are not safe? If arsenic used is in nontoxic organic form then what is the problem, why would the FDA endanger American people? They know what they are doing and who is manipulating who here? Poisoning children with 300 times of allowed arsenic concentrations for what? Profit. The answer is again half-truths. The government does not care about people they just pretend to do until someone exposed them and then it is just industry fault. No, it is not, it is the government fault. Without government approval, nothing can happen. Well at least in the USA. What happens, in this case, is this. When organic arsenic is cooked, cooking alters arsenic profile into arsenite and arsenate. Also, microbes in the chicken manure alter the arsenic into inorganic form as well (Roxarsone and its metabolites in chicken manure significantly enhance the uptake of As species by vegetables. Chemosphere. 2014 Apr;100:57-62). It was shown that more than 96% of Roxarsone added in chicken feed was degraded and converted to arsenite, and other unknown As species. Roots of vegetables could absorb both forms arsenate and arsenite, but only arsenite was transported up to shoots. This study had proved that plants absorb the toxic inorganic As. Transport of arsenic goes like this: Roxarsone in feed › animals › animal manure › soil › crop. Because of all of this "knowledge" the Poison-Free Poultry Act of 2009 was introduced into Congress. Then again the Poison-Free Poultry Act of 2011, then again all of this was a just governmental lie. As a result, in 2013 different groups from environmental movement, agriculture, food safety and public health came together and filed joined lawsuit against the FDA forcing it to respond. In 2015, to avoid public awareness of the entire corrupt system of the FDA, it was forced to withdraw approval for the last of the arsenic-containing drugs keeping this story as quiet as possible. The bad news for the industry is that without the Roxarsone the chicken meat will lose appealing pink color. One more important thing to mention. Chicken manure is used for organic fertilizer production. It can be composted and converted to black gold. Arsenic was still there until 2016.

There are methods of cooking to lower the level in finished rice. The first method is to soak. When you soak the rice it will absorb water but also that will open up the grains structure, so some of the arsenic that is water soluble will leach out from the rice to the liquid. When you soak the rice or beans throw away the water. Do not use it. Also when the rice is cooked some of the arsenic will leach out to the water as well. So again do not let the water evaporate because the arsenic will be still in there. This is the traditional way of cooking. Cook the rice in the proper amount of water and then throw it away. To recap, soak, drain, rinse with fresh water, cook with fresh water and rinse again. Basmati rice tends to contain less arsenic than other types, and brown rice tends to contain more because a big chunk of the arsenic is in the husk. Whit just regular cooking of rice in rice cooker or cooking to dryness without soaking 84% of arsenic will remain. When one part of rice with five parts water is used, only 43% of the arsenic initially detected in the rice will remain. The best method is to soak then rinse then 5 to 1 cooking. That method will eliminate more than 80% of arsenic. And because arsenic occurs naturally, buying organic doesn't generally help. Organic produce consumption does not necessarily impact levels of metals or POPs. If there is arsenic in the soil, it is still "organic" produce.

For marketing purposes, because consumers do not respond well on the words like sewage sludge it has been deliberately renamed as biosolids. The same thing had been done to plain old chicken manure, and it was labeled as "organic" soils and fertilizers even with all of the pollutions coming from the farms. Organic fertilizer must be the good and healthy thing right. Unlike As in organic fertilizer sewage sludge is still there on our plate. When sewage and industrial or municipal wastewater that is full with regular organic excrement but is also filled with other toxic stuff is treated, it will become sewage sludge. It is semi-solid material that is produced as a by-product during sewage treatment in specialized facilities. It is done in stages where primary sludge in created in the primary sedimentation stage and then in a secondary and final sedimentation process after biological degradation, biological sludge that is used as fertilizer is produced. They filter the sewage and let it biodegrade, and then they dry it up and create fertilizer. The properties of secondary sludge can vary depending on the type of biological process that was used.

In most cases, secondary sludge is mixed with primary before treatment and disposal. They are mixed to reduce the overall cost of the treatment plants. One-half of the costs of operating secondary sewage treatment plants can be associated with sludge treatment so by using raw sewage sludge they can reduce the sludge disposal cost significantly. It also gives a significant boost to the phosphorus and nitrogen concentration in the treated fields increasing the growth rate of many crops. The problem with urban sewerage systems is that they have all of the chemicals we use in our homes and many of them are incredibly toxic and do not biodegrade. Also, storm-water runoff from roads and other paved areas, and industrial effluents from all of the manufacturing and other types of businesses and even chemical plants wastewater and so on. It is not just human excrement that goes into sewage sludge like industry people will like us to believe. Sewage sludge will contain organic waste material yes, but will also contain all of the toxic and all of the extremely toxic pollutants used in our modern society. All of them. Sewage sludge will contain, and this had been proven by studies and analysis many types, the viruses, pathogenic bacteria, protozoa, and parasitic helminths, but this is not the big issue because these are all living matter. Sludge treatment and soil-microorganisms and climate can dramatically reduce the number of pathogenic microorganisms, and in time after it has been utilized to the soil, it will pose no hazard. However, if not treated correctly it can give rise to potential hazards to the health of animals that are mostly living on the treated fields but also humans, and plants. In one incident in Walkerton, sewage sludge Escherichia coli and other pathogens contaminated the drinking water supply of this Ontario town.

However, what about toxic chemicals that do not biodegrade? After all of the bioprocesses are over what cannot be eliminated is metals, POPs and other stable chemicals that remain in the soil. Biosolids and farm animals manure plus cannibalistic feed biomagnification just closes the loop for persistent toxins that circle around and because we are at the top of the food chain toxins that come from wild fish and animals, and pollution from environment and all of the new chemicals we annually producing in factories just get added to the loop.

Synthetic fertilizers create many problems too. Fertilizers leach into streams, rivers, lakes and disrupt the balance of aquatic ecosystems. This is creating an excess of nutrients, including nitrogen and phosphorus, in the water. This is food for the sea plants as much as it is food for land grown crops. An abundance of nutrients created by runoff leads to excessive algal blooms. Excessive algal blooms then deplete the water out of oxygen creating oceanic dead zones. Then when these algae start to decompose water quality problem emerge and the result is dead fish and other aquatic organisms. This process is called eutrophication. One of the most significant dead zones worldwide can be found in the Gulf of Mexico, beginning at the Mississippi River delta. This one thing should be enough reason to stop eating anything from the entire ocean at present time. Just this form of imbalance in nature in the form of algae bloom can kill you. I am not kidding. What you do not understand is that these algae are not just some see vegetables that overgrow in seawater from fertilizers runoff and then die off and that it. Some of them or let say most of them are fine and safe and won't do long-term damage except the dead zones, but some of them are not safe because they create and excrete some of the most potent neurotoxins known to man. When they start to overgrow because of all of the nitrogen runoff from the land they bloom and excrete enormous amounts of these neurotoxins to the water. These toxins that are chemically stable do not degrade but start to bioaccumulate like anything else. These toxins do damage in any exposure. If the exposure level is low, they will just worsen overall brain degradation and contribute to brain shrinkage with aging but if the toxins accumulate over the acceptable threshold diseases will appear.

Stephen Hawking is an example of this. Hawking had a form of amyotrophic lateral sclerosis (ALS). ALS is known commonly as Lou Gehrig's disease. ALS is motor neuron degradation disease that in time completely paralyze the patient eventually leading to respiratory failure. It just attacks motor neurons, so the patient's mental capabilities remain intact, and in most cases, death comes after three years when they can no longer breathe on their own. There is no cure for it. ALS strikes previously healthy people seemingly at random. ALS is a progressive disease. That means that it can only go worse over time and usually kills in 2-5 years after first signs of disease. About 10% of people with ALS survive at least ten years. Stephen Hawking was the longest living individual in history with ALS. When ice bucket challenge went viral, many people heard about this disease, and it became a form of a social media awareness campaign that turned into a national phenomenon. Now it is nice to be there for people in need, but that will just pump our own image of self-worth. It would not help to prevent or lower the rate of the disease. Real awareness is something completely different. If people wanted to make the difference and raise awareness, they should do green algae water bucket challenge instead of ice bucket one. ALS is more common than recognized. We have 1 in 400 risks of getting it, and that is in the similar rate level of multiple sclerosis. So let us do some real awareness instead of false ego based one.

In 1944 U.S. forces had recaptured Guam from the Japanese. Initially, United States occupied Guam from Chamorro people on June 21, 1898. And currently, it is under the territory of U.S. It is a small island in the middle of the Pacific Ocean with a big military base. After the war a navy neurologist noticed that local Chamorro people have a high rate of the very deadly form of the strange neurodegenerative disease with symptoms of dementia, shaking, paralysis and death. In some settlements in Guam 1 in 3 people died. The illness was named as amyotrophic lateral sclerosis-parkinsonism/dementia complex (ALS-PDC), known locally as lytico-bodig. They did not know what it is so they just described as amyotrophy (atrophy of the muscles), lateral (from Latin lateralis, meaning to the side) and sclerosis (Greek σκληρός hard) is the stiffening of a structure. The rate of ALS on Guam was 50–100 times the incidence of ALS worldwide. After the systematic exclusion and statistical analysis, it was found that specific seeds of the cycad Cycas micronesica tree in a diet of the local population was the main trigger of the disease. Biochemical analysis associated neurotoxic non-protein amino acid, beta-methylamino-L-alanine (BMAA), as a primary cause of the illness. Cydat trees where suspected because of the use of the seed flour in cooking coupled with reposts of livestock ataxia after eating from it. And indeed BMAA neurotoxin was found in it. The discovery was just a part of research on the disease known as lathyrism. Lathyrism is mostly present in India, China and in the Middle East. It has very similar symptoms like progressive paralysis of the legs. Studies had later linked lathyrism to consumption of certain species of legumes that contained the compound ß-N-oxalylamino-L-alanine (BOAA). The lathyrism was the reason why the researchers tested cycad seeds for BOAA first. When the seed show no concentrations of BOAA very similar substance had been found with a methyl group instead of an oxalyl group—BMAA. So it chemically very similar neurotoxin that just has methyl group instead.

Subsequent studies on rats and monkeys showed the same result in both cases. BMAA is toxic to neurons. However, there was one big difference. Dietary exposure caused immediate symptoms in rats whereas ALS-PDC developed years or even decades after the initial exposure. One other problem was the dose. In the 1980s neurotoxicologist, Peter Spencer did a study and reported the results of paralysis in macaques fed BMAA. However, again the dose used was much higher than the dose that people suffering from ALS were exposed to by cycad flour. People had to eat kilograms of it to ingest a comparable dose. Analysis of BMAA concentrations in cycad seeds by various research groups has highlighted that the toxin was present in the seed at low concentrations. Subsequent investigations confirmed that most of the neurotoxin, around 85 percent was removed from cycad flour during processing. There was a calculation that people would have to eat thousands of kilograms of the stuff every day to get to toxic levels of exposure. In the end, the entire theory was abandoned.

Then in the late 1990s, famed neurologist Oliver Sacks (the one who wrote Awakenings that was adapted into an Academy Award-nominated film in 1990, starring Robin Williams and Robert De Niro) and his colleague Alan Cox made some discoveries and resurrected the BMAA theory. The local Chamorro people by now with knowledge from the research that had been done started to use some tactics as a precaution. They made tortillas from cycad seed flour. However, before they use the seeds, they washed them repeatedly to remove toxins and then gave the water to chickens to drink. If their chickens remained alive after drinking the wash water, the people deemed the seeds safe to grind and eat. However, they also ate other wild animals that they hunted and some of them also feed on cycad seeds as well. For example, for fruit bats and feral pigs, common food was cycad seeds. Oliver Sacks got the idea that it is not the seed that is problematic but the animals that people consume because it is just another case of biomagnification. One of the typical local meals was Mariana flying foxes simmered in coconut cream and eaten whole with skin, bones, brains, and everything. Sacks and Cox in 2002 theorized that these animals that feed on the seeds in time create a neurotoxic reservoir of BMAA in their brain tissues. Because their brains were also eaten on the regular bases by the Chamorros, chronic dietary exposure had created the reservoir of BMAA in their own brain leading after a lag time, to a neuronal meltdown and development of ALS. The consumption of Guamanian flying foxes which fed on the cycads was core to the Chamorro tradition. Also, statistical correlation showed that the decline of the flying fox population due to the excessive hunting correlated with the drop in the number of cases of ALS/PDC presented in Guam. Cox analyzed the skin of preserved museum flying fox specimens (collected five decades previously) and found BMAA concentrations to be extremely high.

The lag time is one of the things that made these diseases hard to track. With leg time people tend to expose them self to the toxin completely without noticing anything wrong and when the pool of this toxin accumulate and disease show the first symptoms, it is already too late. The final closure of the topic was autopsies on the brains of Chamorros that died from ALS/PDC that found high levels of BMAA (A mechanism for slow release of biomagnified cyanobacterial neurotoxins and neurodegenerative disease in Guam Proc Natl Acad Sci U S A. 2004 Aug 17; 101(33): 12228–12231). 13 Canadian subjects had no detectable levels of BMAA. They were just individuals who died of causes unrelated to neurodegeneration. However, when BMAA was measured, it was also found in brains of all of the Canadian patients with Alzheimer's disease. However, wait just a second? These people were in Canada not on Guam. They did not eat flying foxes or Cydat tree seeds.

The real story here is that BMAA neurotoxin was not produced by the tree either. It was produced by Nostoc cyanobacteria, root symbionts of the cycad trees. Bacteria that live in roots of the tree made the toxin. When the toxin gets absorbed by the roots it will be passed to the seeds, then to the bats that feed on them and then to the people. The implication of this scientific discovery is terrifying. If cyanobacteria produce these neurotoxins, it will have massive ramification for public health on a global scale. Cyanobacteria are ubiquitous and can be found in almost every aquatic or terrestrial habitat. They are literary everywhere from damp soil, fresh water, oceans, hot springs, bare rock and soil, rocks in the desert and even Antarctic rocks. The name cyanobacteria comes from the color of the bacteria (Greek: κυανός. Kyanós meaning blue). You know these bacteria as blue-green algae, that blooms from fertilizer runoff.

Cox found the presence of BMAA in most of the variety of cyanobacterial strains tested from all over the globe. It is not just Guam Nostoc strain, it is every strain of this blue-green algae or to be precise 95% of all strains produce BMAA. Because of enormous algae blooms the level of BMAA today needs to be measured and studied. There were studies that have measured the levels of BMAA in some of the higher trophic organisms. High concentrations were detected in various species of fish, mussels, oysters, and plankton thus indicating that the global human population is at high risk of bioaccumulation of this neurotoxic compound through the food chain everywhere in the world.

To this day there is no scientific consensus that BMAA exposure through consumption of contaminated food could play a causal role in various neurodegenerative pathological conditions. In some studies, depending on the methods they did not find BMAA in Alzheimer brain tissue in others they do. Measured levels of BMAA in the brain might not mean causality; proximity is not causality. Some of the most compelling evidence was presented at the International ALS/Motor Neuron Disease (MND) Symposium in 2011. There was research that showed that BMAA is not found in the brain tissue in higher concentrations because it will get incorporated directly into the nerve cell itself. It was shown that BMAA gets incorporated into nerve cell proteins causing the protein misfolding and ultimately cell death. Dunlop and Rodgers reported that the tRNA synthetase enzyme for the amino acid serine mistakenly picks up BMAA thinking that it is serene and then incorporates it into proteins in vitro.

This substance is nothing less than pure mutagen. Consequent auto fluorescence indicated that the proteins misfolded, and the cells died. What we can say for sure is that BMAA might not cause Alzheimer or Parkinson disease just by itself, but it does worsen the condition, and it does cause ALS. Now to fully understand the story of BMAA since many people around the world may be exposed to it we might also ask the question why did some individuals get neurodegenerative effects of it, and some others did not?

Cox suspected that vulnerability may reflect a gene-environment interaction. If this single environmental toxin plays a role in different diseases such as Parkinson disease, ALS, Alzheimer disease and maybe some other diseases as well, this could represent a gene-environment interaction based on individual genetic resilience. However, no one has yet investigated a genetic basis to BMAA vulnerability. It is the same story all over again. Humans did get exposed to this naturally occurring toxin during normal evolution. What is making this disease to increase in prevalence is algae blooms caused by unnatural high levels of nutrient runoff from fertilizer fields, animal waste, sewage, and soil erosion in water that eventually raise the levels of blue-green algae to unnatural high levels. Some people have better genetics dealing with this some might be sensitive. Also it depends on how many seafood you eat. The cause of this disease is not hereditary. It is maladaptation to our current environment. This toxin was found in freshwater fish, saltwater fish, shellfish. Some of the fish have levels of BMAA comparable to those found in fruit bats in Guam. I cannot give estimates here because BMAA concentration varies from a place of sampling. Some species of crab, for example, might be high or low on the toxicity level depending are there algae bloom in the water or not. The more bloom, the more toxin. However, toxins spread everywhere eventually. This could explain the ALS clustering in populations who live around lakes for example. A number of ALS cases have been diagnosed among residents of Enfield, New Hampshire, a town encompassing a lake with a history of cyanobacteria algal blooms. There were six cases of ALS diagnosed from 1975 to 1983 in long-term residents of Two Rivers, in a small Wisconsin community. The probability that this occurred due to chance was less than 0.05%. Cyanobacteria species depending on a type have the ability to produce a different array of metabolites, not just BMAA that are also neurotoxins, hepatotoxins, or dermatoxins. BMAA does not have to kill us to be bad. It can cause neurologic damage and increase the overall toxic load on our bodies and have synergistic effects with mercury and lead and all other neurotoxins to enhance cognitive decline.

In the end, it might not be the only thing that can trigger ALS. BOAA triggers lathyrism for example. It is the same type of neuron death like in ALS. American veterans have more instances in ALS for an unknown reason. The situation in Guam in the last decade or so is promising. Their levels of ALS are significantly lower than in the past, but now they know what the root cause of these neurologic disease epidemic they had to face was. And without the island of Guam rest of the world will still eat seafood thinking that it is health promoting and safe. The problem with nature is that it is hard to science every molecule that exists. There are thousands of natural pollutants like BMAA in nature. Some of them can even be sexually transmitted like ciguatera toxin that again is produced by algae and build up in the food chain, and again it is thermally and chemically stable. It causes nightmares literally with pain and fatigue and burning cold sensation. The reversal of temperature sensation, hot feels as cold and cold feels as hot. It can last for years and in low doses just causes fatigue. The story of a romantic dinner with red snapper in Greek marinade with the wine. Dream tropical paradise vacation turning into cold, painful sex with nightmares. Some of the chronic fatigue syndromes cases are actually ciguatera fish poisoning. In some people, it can cause recurring symptoms during periods of stress, weight loss, exercise or excessive alcohol use even after 25 years of initial exposure. Because all of the pollution most of the fish today have infections both from bacteria and parasites. Never eat raw anything from the water ever in your life. Forget about sushi. Shifts in the balance of nature have consequence. Everything that is unnatural, and when I say that I mean everything that our hominin ancestors did not do or wasn't exposed to is disease promoting with potential for the unknown amount of unidentified toxins. It there were clean and pristine oceans eating predatory fish is still a bad idea and eating a lot of fish is unnatural. Fish is inflammation promoting meat even without all of the pollution.

I am going to provide one additional case of unnatural toxin exposure because it would be impossible to analyze all unnatural toxins that we had created in the Modern Era. It is only essential that we understand logically how our habitat functions so that we can govern our choices with reason and not just with science because science cannot govern our every act. I mentioned the substance named acrylamide in the study of California children and I didn't fully explain what it actually is. Acrylamide is a primarily industrial chemical that has been used in many industrial processes, such as the production of plastics, dyes, and paper. It is additionally utilized in the treatment of wastewater, sewage and the treatment of drinking water as well. It is also found in many of the consumer products, such as some adhesives, food packaging, and caulking. In the US acrylamide is classified as a Group 2A carcinogen and as an extremely hazardous substance. Because of its toxic nature, businesses that have any use of it are subject to strict reporting requirements. In 2002 it was discovered in extremely high concentrations in potato chips and French fries. The concentrations were so high that these two types of food would be banned for children in any normal circumstances. It was also discovered, just not at the same extreme level, but still in the toxic range in all other starchy foods that had been heated higher than 120 °C (248 °F). Such as bread for example. There was no detectable level in foods that were not heated or that were boiled. What happened was that the calculated level of average acrylamide intake was not at the level that posed a risk for negative effects on the nervous system and fertility and from this, it was concluded that acrylamide levels in food were safe regarding the nervous system. However, the synergistic effect that it might have with other environmental toxins were not calculated, or any studies had been done on that subject either. Only concerns were raised on acrylamide human carcinogenicity based on known carcinogenicity in laboratory animals. Rodent studies had associated acrylamide exposure with risk for several types of cancer. Evidence from human studies linked it to kidney cancer, breast cancer, endometrial cancer, ovarian and prostate cancer. So what does the heating do to produce acrylamide? There is amino acid (building block of proteins) named asparagine. It is found in any type of protein including vegetable proteins as well. Some varieties of potatoes have a higher amount of it than any other known food products. When high temperatures start to heat asparagine in the presence of certain starches or sugars, there is a chemical reaction that turns asparagine into acrylamide. To lower the exposure if you care about doing so, you can use low-temperature cooking methods like boiling and microwaving. High-temperature cooking methods, such as baking, frying or broiling, will produce acrylamide depending on the concentrations of the amino acid itself and concentration of starches and temperature and duration of cooking. Longer cooking times increase acrylamide production when the cooking temperature is above 120 degrees Celsius. No animals in nature do things to food as frying. It is an unnatural process, and because it is a new invention concerning evolution, we do not have adequate deface against its toxicity. Once ingested, acrylamide is processed through cytochrome P450 enzyme system and converted into glycidamide and detoxified. Even though our metabolic pathways can help us to detoxify it by some measure, nonetheless, we can still burden our liver detox capability to the level that it will not be able to do its job in time. Eating many chips for example especially if you are a young child can overstress these pathways of detoxification and put you at health risk from excess exposure to this substance. It is possible that our hominin ancestors had been exposed to this chemical because we do have cytochrome P450 enzyme system and Homo erectus may have been roasting some of the starch-rich vegetables, but it is unlikely that they have been exposed to it in the excessive levels as we are today.

Frying destroys molecular consistency of many molecules that are in food. The problem arises when amino acids that are building blocks of our own proteins and cells get damaged. If the damage is partial our bodies will integrate these damaged amino acids into our cells not realizing that they are actually damaged. This will, in consequence, have a mutagenic and cancerogenic effect. Frying and baking also destroy oils that are not thermostable (omega 3 6 9) forcing them to oxidase and to go rancid and cancerogenic too. Some studies show a significant correlation between fried food and some types of cancer. If you have cancer, it would be logical to avoid any food processing except boiling. The list of toxic and cancer-promoting chemicals that can be created in high temperatures is extensive. If you want to avoid acrylamide then no toasted grains, no potato chips, no French fries, no toasted wheat cereals, no cookies and crackers, no roasted grain-based coffee substitutes, no roasted cocoa beans (and chocolate, Nutella and other cocoa made stuff). Some canned black pitted olives can also fall into this higher-risk category regarding acrylamide exposure. Tolerable instances are set to 2,6 micrograms per kilogram of body weight. For a 70kg human, it is 182 micrograms. For children, it is much less than that. And I will argue that the limit is set high deliberately. Setting this limit lower will mean mandatory legal recall of a wide variety of food items we have in our stores and restaurants. McDonald large fries have 82 micrograms. Even at current allowed level, it will be required for example to legally restrict the selling of McDonald large fries to children under 35 kg. If you want to decrease your exposure to dietary acrylamide, you will need to restrict your intake of the above foods. However, again we are forgetting something.

Any food that is fried or baked will have a similar reaction. Not just starchy one. If we eat animal products, the same process will happen just other chemicals will get formed. It is an unnatural activity. I already mention harmane and essential tremor connection. Polycyclic aromatic hydrocarbons (PAHs) and heterocyclic amines (HCAs) are formed when any animal tissue not just muscle meats, no matter from what species, is prepared using high-temperature cooking. Grilling directly over an open flame or pan frying result in the creation of 17 different heterocyclic amines (HCAs). HCAs and PAHs are proven human carcinogens among other things. Heterocyclic describes just the shape but they are still amino acids with damaged molecular structure caused by process of heating and the body does not fully recognize them as damaged. In studies in rodents, feeding them with HCAs resulted in the development of cancers in the couple of different organs including prostate, breast, and colon.

In the lifetime of exposure with all of other toxins and mutagens in an environment adding more is not a good idea. Thousands of different toxins that our liver have to detoxify might not be cancerogenic, but the load itself is what in our new environment is problematic. In clean nature of our past where we evolved in pristine conditions without pollution, our bodies still had to deal with some of the naturally occurring toxins, but we were not overloaded with other chemicals that we are loaded now. Therefore, in our new habitat, we have to think to lower the exposure of every toxin we can because we could not lower them all. However, what we can evade we should, and even toxins that are not deadly should be avoided to lower our overload. Overloaded liver will let some of the more dangerous toxins to accumulate and to do the damage to our cells because it has too much work to deal with, sort of speaking. Going low on the food chain, eating organic, avoiding preservatives, avoiding too much of frying and baking, avoiding natural toxins and drinking clean water is just the start.

Now someone might get the idea that eating raw to avoid this type of toxins like acrylamide and to preserve the phytochemical and antioxidant content is a good choice. Yes, it is, if food is design to be eaten raw by nature itself. Eating raw vegetables is better than cooked but eating raw beans, for example, can kill you. Five raw dried red kidney beans are enough to cause vomiting diarrhea and pain. That is because the substances called lectins, chemicals that paleo diet people find to be one of the root causes of all evil.

To some extent, they can be right. Lectins are a family of proteins that bind to carbohydrates. They are sugar-binding and convert to the glyco portion of glycoconjugates in the cell membranes. The main constituents of human cell membranes include lipids, glycoproteins, lipid-linked proteins, and proteins. So they are in all of us. Lectins are proven to play a different role in cell growth, cell death, body fat regulation, and immune functions. Some of them no one should be consuming ever. However, some of them are necessary. Since plants cannot move, they use their natural chemistry to protect themselves from microorganisms, insects and other animals. One of the defensive chemicals are lectins. They are not to be confused with leptin, which are satiety peptide hormone produced almost exclusively in fat tissue. Lectins play a role in different biological systems. Not just in the human body but also in animals, plants, bacteria, and even viruses. Some are toxic, inflammatory, or both and can have anti-nutrient value. They can block absorption of some nutrients. Some are beneficial and have anti-cancerogenic activity. There is a wide variety of them. Most of them are destroyed by cooking, but some are resistant to cooking and digestive enzymes, but again some of them are destroyed by sprouting. In nature seeds have to stay fresh and ready to sprout so naturally in the seed there are chemicals that will kill all of the putrefying bacteria. These chemicals can be deactivated by soaking, which is the beginning of the sprouting. When the seed starts to sprout it neutralize its protective preservative chemicals that can have ant nutrient and toxic effect.

Avoiding lectins is not possible or almost impossible because they are present in all of our food. They are abundant in raw legumes and grains and in some vegetables, but the more problematic lectins are found primarily in the legumes. Some in wheat can also be problematic. Wheat gliadin, which causes coeliac disease, is a lectin-like substance and it binds to the human intestinal mucosa. Gliadin has been theorized as the coeliac disease toxin for over 20 years. Because we do not digest lectins, they passed into our blood circulation, so we often produce antibodies to them. Everyone has some antibodies to some dietary lectins. The appearance of different lectins can stimulate an immune system response. However, depending on the individual, response can vary. In some individuals, some types of foods can become intolerable after the immune system change or after the permeability of the intestinal line increase so the immune system response will have to increase as well. If we have developed antibodies to them that can be a problem not because of the lectin itself but because of something called molecular mimicry. And that can be a real nightmare. If some chemical gets to our bloodstream and our immune system makes antibody to that chemical and if the chemical is similar to some of our own cells, meaning it has a sequence of amino acids that are the same as the sequence in some of our own cells, then the bad things are going to happen. After cleaning the evil intruder chemical, the antibody will detect our own cell as the same chemical and will attack our own living tissue eating us from the inside. When immune system by mistake of molecular mimicry starts to attack our own cells, the horrors of never curable autoimmune disease begins.

The great news is that lectins are not similar genetically to us because they are from plant kingdom that have different cells then our own and will not cause the autoimmune reactions. However, it still can cause allergies and inflammation. Many lectins are potent allergens. For instance, prohevein is the primary allergen of rubber latex. In recent years, a new strain of genetically modified tomatoes have been created that have added genes for production of prohevein because of its fungistatic properties. Because of this in the future, we can expect a rise in tomato allergies among latex-sensitive individuals. Of specific interest is the fact that lectins can stimulate class II HL antigens on cells that do not usually display them, such as pancreatic islet and thyroid cells. Insulin-dependent diabetes, therefore, can be potential lectin disease. Another possible correlation as a lectin disease is rheumatoid arthritis. In diet-responsive rheumatoid arthritis, one of the most typical trigger foods is wheat. Some of the effects observed in the small intestine in rodents was stripping away of the mucous coat and exposing naked mucosa to abnormal bacteria growth. Lectins also stimulate acid secretion by causing a release of histamine from gastric mast cells. Three central pathogenic constituents for peptic ulcer, stripping away of the mucous defense layer, abnormal bacterial proliferation (Helicobacter pylori), then release of histamine and acid stimulation are all theoretically linked to lectins. However, if we all eat lectins, why don't we all get peptic ulcers, rheumatoid arthritis, and insulin-dependent diabetes? Partially because cells are preserved behind a fine screen of sialic acid molecules and partially because of natural change in the glycoconjugates that coat our cells. However, the sialic acid molecules can be stripped off by the enzyme called neuraminidase, present in several micro-organisms such as streptococci and influenza viruses. This may reveal why diabetes and rheumatoid arthritis tend to occur as a sequence of infections. The best thing to do when you are sick is to listen to your body not your mom and do not eat.

What can happen that is potentially dangerous is the situation when lectins affect the gut wall, and we eat food from the animal kingdom that is genetically similar to our own cells. Lectins can cause inflammation and create damage to the lining of the intestines. If this damage is not regenerated fast enough, the gut can become leaky allowing various molecules (including stuff we do not want) to pass into the bloodstream and that is one of the main factors that are responsible for the creation of autoimmune diseases. Now in the normal situation, lectin inflammation usually is not at the level that is dangerous and should not be the problem but if you have an allergy to some of the lectins, then it might. The brain is the brain, muscle is muscle, sort of speak, so if in the same time we have leaky gut and eat animal tissue, the autoimmune diseases are theoretically possible especially because of our low level of stomach acidity that cannot dissolve animal protein completely. Globular undigested proteins from animal tissue similar to our own tissue entering our bloodstream because of the lectin inflammation in the gut are a recipe for autoimmune diseases. The only thing that is normal is individual amino acids passing thru, if we have more amino acids in the chain in the blood then it is potential invader swimming around and immune system steps into action. For people with leaky gut, Crohn's disease and any type of problem with digestion eating animal protein is in my opinion one leg in the grave. True carnivore with stomach acidity of pH one does not have to worry about this. Also when enough lectins are consumed, it can signal our body to evacuate GI contents. This means vomiting, cramping, and diarrhea. It may further induce a comprehensive immune system response creating inflammation as the body's defenses move in to attack the invaders.

If you eat animal protein or even if you do not, it is a good idea to do allergic testing for every type of food early in the childhood because food allergies can cascade into the leaky gut, then into autoimmune diseases like diabetes type 1 or multiple sclerosis. The worst and the most famous lectin is ricin produced in the seeds of the castor oil plant, Ricinus communis. Ricin was even used in experimental military chemical warfare program during World War 1. There was an attempt to make coating bullets and ricin bombs, but the program did not prove to be particularly useful. It takes precisely 1.78mg of ricin to kill an average adult person. It can even be inhaled. That is about the same amount as few grains of table salt which ricin resembles visually. It is untraceable in toxicology examinations because the poison is just a catalyst that will start a chain reaction in the body. When first symptoms begin to show the ricin is already destroyed and cannot be detected in the body. It is at least ten times more toxic than the most potent nerve gas. A 1% water solution with an explosive burster has the same effectiveness as sarin nerve gas. That is the power of the plants. The only disadvantage ricin has is the time it needs for the victims to die. It will not have the quick tactical effect of nerve gas like sarin if you use it in combat, so it was abandoned as a military weapon. However, for single covert assassinations, it is a useful substance because the assassin can escape long before the first symptoms of poisoning had been detected. Bulgarian dissident Georgi Markov was killed in this way back in 1978 in the middle of the street in London by stabbing him from behind with umbrella. Weaponized umbrella had ricin, and when he was stabbed in the leg with it, it was game over. He died four days later. There is no antidote currently available for ricin poisoning, only some experimental stuff that is not available to the public and not very reliable because the antidote only works while ricin is still in the blood. Usually when the first symptoms start it is already too late. If exposed death is guaranteed. Only vaccination is possible and only is effective for several months by injecting an inactive form of protein chain.

Breaking Bad series actually had inspired several real-life criminal cases involving ricin poisoning. The US government has done everything it can to hide copies for this deadly poison, but in reality, I was able to find one in a couple of minutes. Castor oil seeds contain around 5-10 percent ricin. You just have to remove the oil and fiber and filter it out. Even five to ten raw ground castor seeds will kill an adult human without making the poison. And yes castor oil is perfectly safe, according to the FDA and your grandma, ricin is not in castor oil. When we know about stuff like this, it is easy to spread hysteria about lectins like book Plant Paradox and other bad science made to sell lectin shield products and diets. Also, lectins in the diet are not blood-type specific, so blood type diet is just wrong. It reminds me of the gluten story. Lectin avoidance can become new gluten scam. While many types of lectins are dangerous, there are also health-promoting lectins that can decrease the incidence of certain diseases.

Furthermore, they are necessary for some of the essential biochemical processes in which the body uses lectins to achieve many essential functions, including programmed cell death, inflammatory modulation, and cell to cell adherence. The ones that can cause problems are the ones in beans and if you have food allergies and that is it. Actually low doses of lectins are beneficial by ameliorating obesity, limiting tumor growth and stimulating gut function. Especially for colon cancer. Ricin itself has been under several experiments as a new drug for cancer treatment. There are lectins that kill cancer cells and at the same time don't do anything to normal cells. There are even lectins that force mutagenic cancer cells to go back into regular ones without killing them. The interest started back in 1963 after the discovery that lectins can distinguish between normal and malignant cells. Lectins are so specific that a stool sample can predict the presence of polyps and cancers on bases of lectin binding to the colon lining cells. In a Petri dish, they have so far been able to kill a wide variety of cancers.

Because most of the lectins are in intestines the benefits for colorectal cancer are the highest because most of them will come into contact with colon cells before they are absorbed. Big pharma currently does research on different lectins, and it is expected that in future there will be lectin-based drugs. When we look at studies, dietary consumption of beans has been correlated to lower risk of colorectal cancer, diabetes risk, and mortality from all cases. Consumption of whole grains had been correlated with reduced risk of heart disease, strokes, diabetes, cancer, and mortality from all causes. The same story with other high lectin whole foods. If you are not allergic eating tomatoes or whole grains or beans will actually reduce the overall inflammation in the body even with all of the inflammatory lectins in them. Only legumes are poisonous when raw. So how do we remove the lectins from the beans? If beans are soaked for 5 hours, then 15 minutes of cooking will completely eliminate all lectins in them. If you use a pressure cooker, then time is under 8 minutes. Before the beans are palatable, the lectins would be long gone. If beans are not soaked, then around 45 minutes of pressure cooking will eliminate them but still, they will be palatable after 60 minutes. At any rate, the beans would be free from all lectins if palatable no matter what way we cooked them. One important note, lectins are to some degree resistant to dry heat such as what would occur in baking. Cooking with legume flower that is not soaked and cooked first is not traditional way but also not prudent or smart. The second line of defense against lectins is plain carbohydrates because lectins bind to them instantly. The minor quantities of lectins left after soaking and cooking bind with free carbs in the foods and are effectively deactivated. Only individuals eating a raw diet with certain acute or chronic infections like leaky gut or other conditions may find that lectin minimization is necessary but even in their case it might not be. Lectins are here to stay, but there are some other types of natural toxins besides lectins that we should try to minimize.

There is the whole list of them, and I will mention here just some of the most common ones and ways we could deal with them. Oxalic acid (oxalate) is generally found in spinach (0.3–1.3%), tea (0.3–2.0%), parsley (1.7%) and purslane (1.3%), rhubarb (0.2–1.3%), but may also be found in beans, turmeric, cinnamon, asparagus, broccoli, collards, lettuce, celery, cabbage, cauliflower, turnips, beets, peas, coffee, cocoa, potatoes, berries, and carrots. Oxalates are also present in most of the fruits and vegetables in usually small amounts. However, some of the vegetables have them in large amounts. Oxalic acid has the ability to bind to calcium creating calcium oxalate and also to other minerals as well as decreasing the nutrient value of the food by decreasing the bioavailability of minerals. Oxalate also plays a role in the formation of kidney stones. About 65 percent of kidney stones consist of calcium oxalate. For individuals with kidney stones or kidney problems, high oxalate food should be avoided. That will include turmeric. If someone already has kidney problems, he or she should really watch their intake of turmeric. Cinnamon and turmeric actually contain about the same amount of oxalates but with one big difference. Oxalates in turmeric are soluble (readily absorbed) in around 90 percent range. For people with kidney problems that are prone to the formation of the stones, the upper limit is one teaspoon of turmeric per day. Oxalates are a form of antinutrient. One of the primary concerns about oxalate is that it can bind to some of the minerals in the gut. That will prevent the body from absorbing them. Because they can bind calcium and other minerals spinach for example and beet greens are therefore poor sources of calcium. If we take a look into toxicity, it has been estimated that for 59kg human a lethal dose of oxalic acid is 22g. Spinach has one of the most abundant levels of oxalic acid, 0.97 g per 100-gram serving. Theoretically, it is possible to eat enough spinach to die. You would need to eat 3 kg of spinach to consume the 29.1 g of oxalic acid. Oxalate is insoluble in water so cooking would not remove it. It is complicated to remove from food so don't overeat on spinach. Actually many foods that have oxalate are very health promoting and avoiding them completely is not necessary. Oxalate deprived diet is only necessary option for people with kidney stones. Some of the oxalates can be broken down by probiotic bacteria in the gut. However, some people do not have healthy microbiome, and antibiotics decrease the number of probiotic bacteria. Studies have found that individuals with inflammatory bowel disease have an increased risk of developing kidney stones. It had also been shown that oxalate levels are found in urine in patients who had any type of surgeries that alter gut function, for example, gastric bypass surgery. It is important to eat healthy and have good microbiome in the first place. For any individual that suffers from any kind of gut dysfunction or if you are taking antibiotics a low-oxalate diet might have a health benefit. If you are in that category, you can always choose vegetables at low levels like kale. There are merely 2 milligrams of oxalates in a cup of kale.

Phytic acid (also known as phytate) is detected in bran and germ of various plant seeds and in grains, legumes, and nuts. Why many people have a problem with phytate-rich foods is because phytic acid by itself is a source of phosphorus, but it is also a very good chelator of magnesium, iron, copper, calcium, and zinc. Because phytate-rich vegetables are absorbed at a slower pace and provide moderate plasma glucose responses than foods that do not contain phytate. It has been theorized that phytate could have a therapeutic role in the management of diabetes. It also may have utility as an antioxidant. So it has many of the beneficial traits, but it also has the ability to cause essential mineral deficiencies. The recommendation is to remove it. It is heat stable but can be removed by fermentation or soaking. Highest phytate levels are measured in soy. For soybeans, it takes a long period of fermentation or soaking to make a meaningful reduction. Commercial soy milk is not soaked before making because of the lipoxygenase enzyme in soy that needs to be deactivated by blanching whole soybeans before grinding, or the soymilk will have a grassy taste to it.

There are also chemical substances in certain raw foods that can suppress and interfere with the thyroid gland uptake of iodine. If you have a goiter or marginal iodine intake and most regular people do not take enough of iodine because they do not eat sea vegetables, you will have to lower the consumption of goitrogens (glucosinolates). Goitrogenic foods include soybeans, spinach, sweet potatoes, peanuts, cassava, pears, peaches, and strawberries. Also, the entire vegetable group of the Brassica genus is goitrogenic, and that group includes cabbage, broccoli, mustard greens, cauliflower, Brussel sprouts, radishes, canola, and rapeseed. Goiter has also been associated with the consumption of large quantities of uncooked cabbage or kale. There is no iodine in the land. It is washed away by water, thus all of it ends up in oceans. Land vegetables cannot produce iodine because there is none in the earth. Only sea vegetables can pick it up from the ocean, or you will have to take an iodine supplement. I personally do both.

Also, my recommendation is to avoid all oil, but if you have to use it, then there are oils that you need to avoid especially. For example, widespread use of rapeseed oil began in the 1940s and 50s. In rodent studies feeding rapeseed oil to rats was correlated with lipidosis in the cardiac tissue with significantly increased levels of cholesterol. Cardiac problems such as thickening of the epicardium, increased fibrous tissue in different areas of the myocardium are just one side effect. There are also growth retardation and mortality. There is an acid in the rapeseed oil called erucic acid that was identified as the primary causative agent. Because the rapeseed oil is so cheap to produce the industry back in the 1970s created rapeseed oil variant without erucic acid. It is canola, a type of rapeseed with oil that contains reduced levels of erucic acid. In 1995 Monsanto created GMO version of canola oil that is used today everywhere because it is the cheapest of the oils to produce. It is added to food products left and right. Canola oil produces a pretty mild taste so that it can be used or mixed in everything especially with more expensive oils like olive oil. When you go to the restaurant, and you see a bottle of olive oil on the table guess what. It is not. Restaurants use cheap canola oil to blend with more expensive olive oil so that they can save money and because the canola oil is mild the blend of canola-olive oil will still look and taste like olive oil. Cooking oil in almost all of the professional kitchens is usually a mix of 75% canola 25% olive oil. If you ask them what cooking oil they use, what do you think the answer will be? Usually they will say that resonant only use extra virgin olive oil. No, they do not. They use GMO canola oil. Limit for the erucic acid in Canola oil by the FDA standards has to be lower than 2 percent but again it is dose-dependent. If you use a lot of canola oil even that 2% might have an adverse health effect. So why use it at all? Supporters of the canola oil paint the picture that it is one of the healthiest oils on the planet because it is rich in omega 3s, low in saturated fats and is a good source of oleic acid. Now, who do you think is pushing this marketing propaganda? Plant-based omega 3s are so unstable that they will go rancid in a matter of hours when exposed to oxygen. Even if you want to eat omega three rich flaxseed, grind it up an eat it immediately, and never buy any refined omega three rich oil in the bottle. Then I will also ask another question. Why eat any oil at all for that matter? Oil is just a refined empty calorie without any nutritional value.

When we look at the fruits, there are some toxins even there. Citrus fruits and grapefruit especially produce a variety of different chemicals in their peels that may have adverse interactions with drugs. Typically, Citrus fruit juice is usually produced with the whole fruit, including the peel, so my advice is, don't by commercial grapefruit juice and make your own.

Another substance Safrole that s found in nutmeg, cinnamon, camphor, and sassafras oil is confirmed to be a human carcinogen. Before FDA ban of it in 1960, it was used to flavor root beer and other foods. Root beers are now artificially flavored as a result of the FDA ban. At a concentration of 1% in the diet, it can produce testicular atrophy, bone marrow depletion, weight loss and malignant liver tumors in rats.

One other poison is in nutmeg, myristicin. It is a naturally occurring insecticide. It is also present in parsley, carrot, black pepper, celery, and dill but not as much concentrated level as it is in nutmeg. Myristicin produces a low monoamine oxidase inhibitor action and by elemicin may be metabolized to an amphetamine-like substance that has hallucinogenic effects similar to lysergic acid diethylamide (LSD). The dose level of 6–7 mg/kg, may cause psychotropic effects, such as euphoria, increased alertness, freedom and a feeling of irresponsibility. Unpleasant symptoms, such as the feeling of impending doom, anxiety, tachycardia, tremor, fear are also being reported. Symptoms ordinarily follow three to eight hours window after ingestion and resolve within a day or two. Sometimes nutmeg is used as a recreational drug especially in the time of hippie culture and in prisoners, drug addicts, and college students. However, the most common and medicinal use of nutmeg during the history is as an abortifacient. The reason abortion is legal is not because the woman rights movement to kill babies won the political battle, but because the government wanted to have some sort of control. Mothers in entire human history had always kill their own babies if the baby did not fit the mother's interest. Nobody was able to stop that practice because the woman just has to take some nutmeg and don't tell anyone about it. In Ancient times and in the Middle Ages, it was common practice. The ancient Greek town of Cyrene at one time had the entire economy based on the production and export of the powerful abortifacient plant Silphium. Silphium export was so important to the local business that it even appeared on coins minted there. In the Middle Ages in Europe the Catholic Church inquisition targeted people who dispensed abortifacient herbs as witches and often persecuted them in witch-hunts. In English law, abortion had become legal in 1803 and before that, it was the same story. Woman killed their babies with different kinds of drugs. Women who took drugs for abortions would describe their actions as "bringing on a period" and "restoring the menses." One of the drugs used was nutmeg. At the normal concentration present in food toxicity arising from myristicin is low, but it is still a toxic substance that is better to avoid.

In potatoes, there are natural pesticides that are produced the glycoalkaloids, solanine, and chaconine. The most significant concentrations are in the peels, sprouts, and sun-greened areas. Synthesis of chaconine and solanine is stimulated by aging, mechanical injury, potato beetle infestation, and light. If potatoes get exposed to light in the marketplace or in the field, they can turn green, and that will lead to glycoalkaloid concentrations that can be unsafe for human consumption. Green or blighted potatoes can have to about seven-fold concentrations of solanine. There is no evidence that solanine and chaconine are carcinogenic in animals or humans, but it is a toxic substance, so my advice is to avoid green potatoes.

Many foods like cereals, oilseeds, spices and three nuts, rotten fruits, and vegetables can be contaminated with mycotoxins (aflatoxin, ochratoxin A, patulin, fusarium) produced by fungi. Fungi produced toxins can be very potent and able to cause severe damage to the nervous system, kidneys, and liver but they are mutagenic and carcinogenic at the same time. Mycotoxins are not biodegradable, cannot be destroyed by freezing or cooking and can circle around in the food chain starting from the infected feed crops. We can find them in dairy and meat. The most potent mycotoxins aflatoxin is commonly found in peanuts because the peanuts are attacked by the strain of fungi that produce it. It can also be hidden in some other foods of tropical origin, but the peanuts are the most infected. There is no way to reduce your exposure to mycotoxins, only one is to avoid foods that are not, or don't appear fresh.

All raw mushrooms have toxins too. Mushrooms have very tough cell walls made of chitin, a material that is not digestible if you do not cook them and are grown in manure fertilizers. The manure is generally sterilized before use, but it is still a vibrant medium for bacterial growth if the sterilization process is not done correctly. The typical white mushroom also contains a number of potentially toxic substances, such as agaritine, a derivative of glutamic acid (the most abundant amino acids in the human body). Agartine was proven to be carcinogenic in mice although studies on humans lack it is still a suspected carcinogen. As agaritine is not heat-stable, heating mushrooms reduce the potential risk.

The big message here is to focus on variety. Your body can absolutely handle trace amounts of natural toxins in foods, but if you eat the same stuff over and over again, for example, you are the kid that eats chips every day, it will build up and create a toxic load. Thing as innocent as licorice can kill you. When licorice is consumed in large amounts, it may be harmful. For example, in one reported case there where hypokalemia leading to cardiac arrest. A 58-year-old woman died because she had been eating about 1.8 kg of licorice per week. This licorice has an effect on the body to lose potassium and organism could become potassium deficient (dubbed "glycyrrhizism" after glycyrrhizic acid). Hypokalemia clinically have symptoms of sodium retention and edema with severe hypertension, cardiac arrhythmias, alkalosis, and muscular symptoms. If you are already potassium deficient 100 g licorice per day is all you need to give you the first signs of hypokalemia. So be smart and use common sense and focus on a variety of whole organic foods.

There are a couple of other ways where we can try to lower our toxic load. Natural chemicals like lectins are something that is here to stay, but there is another line of actions we can take. First, we can start with most basic stuff like the water we drink. If we cannot escape chemicals in our food, we can try to eliminate them from the water we drink. The CDC considers fluoride as one of the ten public health achievements of the 20th century. It is viewed as a triumph over tooth decay. Today most of the toothpaste sold contains fluoride and 72% of all water in the US is fluoridated. The first use of fluoride was for the eradication of vermin and ever since it was a crucial ingredient in rat poison and insecticides. At early days of fluoride use, it was only known as poison not just for men, but for the environment as well. It was a crucial ingredient in the Manhattan project and nuclear weapons too. It was added in Auschwitz water supply and water of Siberian gulags for his effect on the human mental state. It is hazardous waste from phosphate fertilizer industry which cannot be dumped into the streams or sea by international law and cannot be used locally because it is too concentrated. I will analyze the real history behind industry and fluoride use in the second part of the book series so that we can try to help ourselves and be smart. However, there are other pollutants in tap water that water plants do not test like inorganic metals and microplastic fibers (83% of the samples were contaminated worldwide), and other nanoparticles that we cannot measure.

When a substance is in the nanometer range what that actually means is that the substance is small enough to penetrate a cell and that means it can penetrate all organs including the brain. There are some studies done, and it has been proven that microplastic has an effect on wildlife but human studies are not here yet. Microplastics have the ability to absorb toxic chemicals as well, and research on wild animals shows that they are released in the body. Microplastic was also found in a few samples of commercially bottled water tested in the US. The problem is that they cannot exceed safety levels because there are none. No safety level regulation, only guidelines. Ever hear of trihalomethanes (TTHMs), which are linked to bladder cancer, skin cancer, and fetal development issues and hexavalent chromium made notorious by the film Erin Brockovich or Radium-226 and Radium-228. All of these contaminants I just mention always had been detected above legal guidelines.

For hundreds of other contaminants, the government does not impose any requirements at all. One of the most prevalent toxins such as perchlorate and PFOA/PFOS (chemical cousins of Teflon) occur in millions of Americans tap water. Because the EPA does not regulate them, they do not show up in any statistics. Sensitive groups of people, like pregnant women and children, are at higher risk for health complications, especially from the list of following contaminants that are regularly detected in tap water like lead (this is a bigger problem in towns with older water systems), and atrazine (endocrine-disrupting substance is one of the most regularly detected pesticides in US waters) and vinyl chloride (used to make PVC plastic products). I will not list all of the detected pollutants it would be a long read. Logically in my mind, only clean water and the only water that I use for cooking and drinking is distilled water. Now be warned this is a double-edged sword at the same time.

Dealing with demineralized water can have adverse effects too. It is not something average people should do if they do not completely understand the entirety of the process first. How many people know that distilled water does not conduct electricity? It even has a different magnetic charge potential than hard water. Also, it is not unnatural. All clouds in the world are distilled water. Rain and snow too. It is not some chemical produced in the lab like Coca Cola. It is just the pure water H2O without anything else in it. Water purification is a big business especially in countries that do not have clean sources. More than a billion people even to this day drinks filthy water and do not have any form of sanitation. Diarrhea to this day due to the poor sanitation kills an estimated 842,000 people every year globally. By 2025, 1.8 billion people are projected to be living in regions with absolute water scarcity. Water is big business, and the business will grow. On the other hand, water is one of the contributing factors to our toxic overload. People who are in the business of water often don't do good science and are more interested in profit. Another thing is that what has influenced the field of water science and technology of purification is a lot of new age philosophy. From normal glucose metabolism, half the oxygen molecules in CO2 that you exhale is from water not from the air. You cannot use the oxygen in the water for respiration but it is still oxygen, and your body needs it for other things. There is much misinformation about detoxifying properties of water and distilled water in particular.

In the human body the water functions as a solvent and a medium for the transport of nutrients. It is also a transport mechanism for waste products. It regulates body temperature, lubricants the joints and has many other biochemical reactions. It is the water, only water H2O not any other dissolved and suspended minerals that do any of these functions. It is just water. When water is low in TDS (total dissolved solids) that means that it has not too many dissolved minerals in it. If water is distilled, that means that it does not have anything in there but H2O. Total dissolved solids in distilled water are zero. It also has different electrical charge properties that makes distilled water unique in that manner that it has a capability to attract inorganic minerals and toxins just by itself. Distilled water wants to saturate itself sort of speak, and that is a property that can be wary useful if you want to detoxify yourself. It is believed that distilled water can help cure arthritis by washing out excess calcium and other inorganic minerals from deposits in joints and other parts of the body. There is a big difference between inorganic and organic minerals. Realistically, minerals are just inorganic metals, so it makes no difference where you get your minerals. The most important factor when we talk about organic vs. inorganic minerals is not composition, it is the same metal, but it is the size and the form they are in. A plant takes the artificial, inorganic minerals from the soil where it is growing that are big chunks of metal if you like that analogy. When plants take up inorganic minerals from the ground by the roots then they synthesize them, or if you like break them down into a molecular size and form that are small enough to do regular biological functions in the living matter. Mineral water comes from the stream is saturated with inorganic molecules. The size of this minerals is not small enough for us to do biological functions so we call them inorganic, not because they are some other molecular substance but just because the size of the molecule is too big. Think of it this way, in mineral water coming from the streams there are also small chunks or rocks that water brake off, but you cannot see them with the naked eye. They are small but not small enough, at least not small enough to be used as an organic form of minerals. There is only one way that the human digestive system can break down larger tightly bound minerals into usable ions, and that is with the stomach acid. The food transit time through the stomach is about one hour. If the inorganic mineral ion is not ionized during this small amount of time and mineral moves from the high acid environment of the stomach no further beneficial breakdown will take place in the small intestines. All further break down ceases. If the inorganic mineral compound is already relatively small like from deep spring water, it might get degraded to smaller monoatomic scale particles by acid in the stomach and be bioavailable. Once minerals left the acidic environment of the stomach the remainder of the non-ionized minerals are no use for us and are in no way available to do any biological functions inside our body except negative ones.

Usually, they will just pass through our GI tract unusable. But If you ingest big chunks of metals called inorganic minerals they might end up in the bloodstream in small quantities. However, they can pass into the bloodstream in the large quantities if you have leaky gut or inflammation in intestines. They will not be small enough to integrate into cells or do any other biological function and will create deposits in the body if the body does not remove them out.

There is unproven speculation that you will even receive from your regular MD that distilled water is dangerous for your health because it would leech minerals out of the body and can cause some of the mineral deficiencies. Speculation is that absorbing extremely purified water, treated by distillation, reverse osmosis, or deionization, leaches minerals from the body. Because there are minerals in the water at the first place drinking distilled water will make problems it the same manner as removing for example husk from the wheat with all of its minerals and eating just refined flour. They say that minerals in water are a necessary part of our mineral absorption. There were some Russian studies done on this topic and are available through the World Health Organization. The summary was that fluid and electrolytes are better replaced with water containing a minimum of 100 mg/L of TDS. However, this only has relevance in specific situations where the human body was exposed to heavy exertion and sweating. It is the market for sports drinks and there is only one substance glucose, regular sugar, that was added to help muscles to replenish the loss of glycogen quickly and to promote more energy in prolonged exercise. Low TDS or demineralized water has nothing to do with it, and for everyday drinking and cooking purposes, it is the best choice. The body has the mechanisms to regulate within very narrow limit the concentrations of minerals (ions) and water as well in all cells and all organs in the body. The organ that is most responsible for mineral balancing is kidneys. They maintain ion concentrations and not just sodium and potassium and calcium but most of the minerals in the normal range during a process of elimination and reabsorption.

There is process called osmosis or osmotic pressure. When sodium ions outside of the cell and potassium ions inside of the cell are out of balance, then the osmotic pressure is out of balance. That will cause the water to flow across the cell membrane to neutralize the difference in osmotic pressure. Any changes that can happen in a reasonable range of concentration of ions is adjusted in a couple of seconds because water moves quickly through cell membranes. Drinking distilled water (0 to 100 mg/L TDS) has nothing to do with it. If any changes occur in the body, it will be rapidly brought to equilibrium with absolutely no consequence. It is the kidneys that in reality control the overall concentration of the constituents of body fluids and not some minuscule amounts of inorganic minerals in tap water. Kidneys in average men filter about 180 liters of water per day. Over 99% is reabsorbed to the bloodstream, and only 1.0 to 1.5 liters are eliminated as urine. If you drink distilled low ion concentration TDS water, nervous and hormonal feedback mechanisms will cause the kidneys to eliminate extra water that is not needed and thus maintain the ion concentration in the body fluid to normal values. The opposite is also true. If the ion concentration in the fluid to be filtered is higher than normal, kidneys homeostatic mechanism will keep fluid osmolality normal by retaining water.

That is why you bloat when eating too much salt and too little potassium. It is not the sodium that is a problem. It is unopposed sodium because there is a lack of potassium in the body. When a healthy person drinks low TDS water, it should not cause any health issues. Significant nutritional deficiencies might cause a leaching problem in the long run, is a what MD will argue. How much of consuming one to two liters of low TDS water on a daily basis cause a leaching problem in reality? We will have to look into this with more detail. If we count all of the minerals in spring water as organic, they will not be able to compound to more than a couple of percent of total minerals digested. Usually, minerals should come from food, not from water. Drinking pure, pristine spring water from unpolluted earth of the past it would not be a problem. Now it is. And distilled water may have some benefits too. WHO had done experiments on volunteers. Results showed that when people start to drink distilled water, the increased diuresis happens with 20% more body water volume, and also serum sodium concentrations decreasing. So you excrete more water and lose some sodium. The second thing that was observed was the decrease in potassium serum concentration. To sum it up, drinking distilled water increase elimination of sodium, potassium, chloride, calcium and magnesium ions from the body. Distilled water interacts with another gastrointestinal tract by osmoreceptors, causing an enhanced movement of sodium ions into the intestinal lumen. This will then cause a slight reduction in osmotic pressure in the blood with the following enhanced discharge of sodium into the blood as an adaptation response. In response volume receptors in the bloodstream are activated, inducing an increase in sodium elimination. Now, this will not be a problem in nature, but especially now it is not because we have our salt shaker on every table and this can be actually beneficial depending on how much salt you eat and how much of distilled water you drink.

There is one other and real issue with demineralized water, and that is why I said you need to know what you are doing. When used for cooking, soft water was found to leech a substantial amount of minerals out of food no matter what that food is. In some cases, losses can reach up to 60 to 90 percent. Numbers for calcium and magnesium are about 60 percent, manganese 70 %, copper 66 %, cobalt 86 % and so on. This can represent a problem because if you cook with soft or distilled water and then throw away that water, you are going to lose much of nutrition. That is why you do not cook with it if the water that is used for cooking is not going to be consumed. When you soak beans, for example, use regular water. When you cook beans use regular water or when you cook anything that is going to be rinsed after use regular water.

In contrast, distilled water capability to leech nutrients from food is turned into a positive thing if you are going to drink that water. When we eat, we do not absorb all of the nutrients that are in food. We absorbed some of them, but some of them are not absorbed. It is what we absorbed not what we eat sort of a thing. So using soft or distilled water can help us to absorb more from the food. For example, use it to make tea. Or when I want to make a soup or some other dish, I use distilled water because it will leach from the food and help me get more from the same food than regular water and I know it would not have all the polluting chemicals in there. When I eat that soup or drink tea, it is not distilled water anymore. If I want to make soy milk, for example, I am going to use the knowledge of water to my benefit by soaking the beans in regular water and then cooking the beans in regular water that will not leach much of the nutrients from the beans. However, then when I want to blend them into the milk, I will rinse the beans and use distilled water for blending because I want to leech most of the nutrients from the beans to make the milk. So again you need to know what you are doing. I personally don't drink much of the water because I drink a lot of vegetable juices through the day and I eat a lot of fruits that are mostly water and plus all the water from cooked meals, so I do not have leaching problem. I like the cleanness and leaching potential of distilled water for detoxification, but again I will drink no more than maybe glass or two in the day. If you drink 2 liters of water because you do not eat fruit or vegetables and don't eat cooked meals and are already potassium deficient like 98% of Americans and then go on a diet with gallons of detoxifying distilled water you might get into a more deficient state then the one you are already in. So again I cannot tell you to drink or not to drink it, it is a more complex issue, and you need to do your own research based on the quality of the mineral content of your diet.

Why I drink and cook with it is precisely because of its potential to leach toxins and inorganic minerals out, and regular minerals I get from food or even some time supplements depending on my diet. I usually take iodine and some organic trace minerals solution from time to time. One more thing on leeching minerals. It will not leach any minerals that have already become integrated into the cells. It collects only minerals that have already been rejected or excreted by the cells. Mostly inorganic minerals that have a different electrical charge then organic and that are themselves attracted to the distilled water by the charge. Distilled water will not leach minerals from your tissue cells. I do periodic blood testing to see the levels of electrolytes and other minerals, and I never had a problem. However, again that is me. I do not do anecdotal stories about leeching, I do self-experimentation and test everything.

And one more thing that is important. Some chemicals are not water soluble. This form of fat-soluble toxins body cannot eliminate through urine. It must be eliminated through the fiber in the intestines. Fiber is our natural detoxifier for fat-soluble chemicals. Detoxifying without fiber is not complete. The best thing to detoxify is something that has distilled water, all the minerals and vitamins, and fiber. So you can try to do distilled water fasting with psyllium husk and organic mineral solution or just eat a lot of raw organic vegetables and keep in mind that detoxification also depends on the half-life of the substances you have already ingested. Distillation does not remove all of the toxins also. Toxins that can be turned into vapor below 100 degras Celsius will be distilled with the water. These are usually some of the pesticides. They can be removed and often home distillatory devices have secondary filter made from carbon just because of this. Also, radioactive particles will not vaporize because they have a higher boiling temperature than water. For people who live in the Fukushima area and for all preppers out there to know that when nuclear winter comes you can distill the water and it will lose all of the radioactivity.

There are many health talks about the benefits of "ionized water" or "alkaline water." It is possible that water contains dissolved ions. Meaning some metallic atoms or electrically charged molecules that can transfer electricity. Ideally, distilled pure water is nothing more than just H2O molecules, and that is it. These H2O molecules are arranged and linked together in free and chaotic network structure with individual molecules bumping into one another all the time. Water in its liquid form is not a geometrical and arranged structure like ice. Water molecules also show a very slight affinity to dissociate (ionize) into hydrogen and hydroxide ions: H2O; H + + OH-. The level of this is minuscule because the opposite reaction is much stronger in bringing back the status quo instantly. On average only about two in one billion of molecules of H2O are dissociated.

No technological process or chemical additive is capable of increasing these ion concentrations in pure water. Pure water can be regarded to be ion-free, as evidenced by the fact that it will not conduct an electric current. There is no known technological method or chemical additive that is able to increase these ion concentrations in pure water above these two in one billion minute levels. These levels are so small that for most realistic and practical purposes pure water can be considered ion free. Distilled water has no ions, as shown by the fact that it is unable to conduct electric current.

Acidic and alkaline water has nothing to do with the water at all, and that is what people need to understand. All water contains both H + ions and OH- ions. If the amount of H + exceeds that of OH-, the water is acidic. If there are more OH- ions than H +, the water is alkaline. If the pH values are lower than seven water is acidic, alkaline solutions are more than 7. Pure distilled water, has no ions and that means that the distillation can never be alkaline or acid, nor can it be produced by electrolysis. Since alkaline liquid always has an excess of OH ions, it must also always contain another type of positive ion in addition to H + to compensate for the opposite charges. This additional positive ion is almost always a metallic ion such as magnesium, calcium or sodium. Similarly, acidic water must always contain negative ions in addition to OH-. This means that waters whose pH differs from 7 are never pure in the chemical sense. Distilled water is pure and can never be alkaline or acidic. Groundwater containing different metal ions that it picks up such as calcium and magnesium can be made slightly alkaline by electrolysis, but that does not mean anything. As soon as "healthy alkaline" water enters the stomach and it is mixed with highly acidic gastric fluid in the stomach, its alkalinity disappears.

The idea that we should consume alkaline water to neutralize the effects of acidic foods is not correct and not just that, it is a very bad idea as well. By exhaling carbon dioxide, our bodies will get rid of excess acid. It is not a big of a problem. However, if you really do de-acidify your stomach, it will cause the problem of successful protein degradation and will interfere with digestion. If acidity in the stomach is lowered by any means during the meal, it will mean that food will not be digested properly. There are benefits only for people with acid reflux (Potential benefits of pH 8.8 alkaline drinking water as an adjunct in the treatment of reflux disease. Ann Otol Rhinol Laryngol. 2012 Jul;121(7):431-4.). This study have founded that alkaline water with pH 8.8 does instantly denature pepsin, rendering it permanently inactive. So for the patients that have reflux disease alkaline water can help in acid-buffering capacity and may have therapeutic benefits. However, if you do not have reflux, drinking it during or after the meal will cause the lowering of the acid level in the stomach and interfere with food degradation and interfere in the nutrient absorption. If you want to drink it, then do not drink alkaline water except on an empty stomach. Supporters of drinking alkaline water still believe in its many proposed health benefits, like detoxifying properties, immune system support, colon-cleansing, weight loss, cancer resistance, anti-aging properties, hydration, skin health, and the list goes on and on.

There are actually the couple of Chinese studies that discovered some of the health benefits in a form on anti-oxidative support (Alkaline Ionized water enhancing heat tolerance and anti-oxidative function of heat-exposed mice. Department of Military Hygiene, the Second Military University, Shanghai 200433, China). The conclusion was that alkaline ionized water could enhance heat tolerance of heat-exposed mice and it might be related to enhancing anti-oxidative function against the damage by free radicals. This was a surprise to me, but I do not believe that the Chinese People's Liberation Army would do a bad science experiment. Chinese did a couple of studies. In this study (Preliminary observation on changes in blood pressure, blood sugar and blood lipids after using alkaline ionized drinking water First Hospital of Shanghai Textile, Shanghai 200060, China) they did find something even more interesting. The objective was to analyze the changes in blood sugar, blood pressure, and blood lipids in patients with diabetes mellitus, hyperlipidemia, and essential hypertension. After they have drunk alkaline ionized water the blood lipids and blood pressure levels dropped in some subjects even to the normal ranges. The study concluded that ionized alkaline water might be used as one of the accessory therapeutic methods for diabetes mellitus, hyperlipidemia and essential hypertension. One more study (Effects of alkaline Ca~ (2+)-water on blood pH, calcium level and immune function in rats School of Life Science, South China Normal University, Guangzhou 510631, China) discovered that alkaline water did not significantly influence the blood pH and calcium concentration but did enhanced the immune function in rats significantly.

What is going on? It bugged me. There are two types of alkaline water. The artificial alkaline water which is generally tapped water run through an electrical ionizer to make the pH more alkaline and bottled spring or mineral water. Naturally-occurring mineral water contains alkalizing compounds in the form of rocks that it picks up, such as magnesium, silica, calcium, bicarbonate, and potassium. You can also purchase ionizing water machines. Water ionizers are the machines designed to work as water electrolyzes but what they do in reality is just to use platinum or titanium to make water alkaline. They do not add any of the minerals found naturally in the ground. You can just ad backing soda for cheap, and you will have alkaline water, but why does it matter at all. When electrolysis or if you like the electrochemical process split water molecules to form hydrogen and oxygen by an electric current the two types of substances will be created and none of them will be the real water. "Water" near the cathode would be alkaline and "water" near the anode would be acidic. Water ionizers work by simply siphoning off the water near the cathode that has higher pH (i.e., be more alkaline) and water near anode would have increased levels of H+ making it acidic. With machines like Kengen, you do not drink true alkaline water made in nature. They are lying to you; it is one more scam. You are actually drinking regular tap water with added hydroxide ions making it alkaline. It is not water at all. It just looks like water, but it is filled with hydroxide ions created by electrolysis. People talking about antoxidative properties of this kind of Kengen created hydroxide ions filled water usually forgot or don't even know the answer to one very important question. What happens after that hydroxide (OH–) that is antioxidant donate its electron? What happens is that it became one of the most cytotoxic oxygen radical: the hydroxyl radical. Hydroxide is not an antioxidant, no matter what someone tells you. Hydroxide (OH–) is higher in alkaline water, but it is not a biological antioxidant. Hydroxyl radicals can occasionally also be produced as a byproduct of immune system activation. Macrophages and microglia (a type of immune cells) generate this compound to fight against some types of bacteria. The destructive action of hydroxyl radicals has been implicated in several neurological autoimmune diseases and can damage virtually all types of macromolecules. I will not personally take any antioxidant no matter how powerful it is if it has the potential to turn itself into free radical. Read the sentence above again and memorize it well. The hydroxyl radical has high reactivity and a very short in vivo half-life of 10 seconds. This makes it a very toxic substance to the organism. Unlike superoxide, which can be detoxified by superoxide dismutase, the hydroxyl radical cannot be eliminated by an enzymatic reaction and once created it will do full damage. Our bodies never have to deal with this molecule in the past. It is new and non-natural antioxidant that has the potential to do a lot of damage if not eliminated from the body. And that is the real issue. Our bodies have no enzyme to eliminate them. Never drink Kangen Water Machine fake alkaline water filled with hydroxide ions created by electrolysis.

There are some real benefits from real alkaline water, and that benefit is hydration. It took me long time but eventually I found the different line of research studies and I understood what is the science behind positive effects of alkaline water found in those studies done in China. Water molecules stick together in clusters. In a normal conditions water molecules arrange themselves in clusters of 14 molecules. When electrolysis breaks the bonds between oxygen and hydrogen creating hydroxide (antioxidant) and hydrogen ions it also brakes down clusters to the smaller size. Also in alkaline water, these clusters can be as small as five water molecules. They make the water a better solvent and increase fluidity. The reason why boiling water has lower surface tension is that of this smaller clustering of water molecules. If water gets too much energy as heat, it loses the clustering ability completely and became a monoatomic form of water know as steam. And I think this is where some of the benefits of alkaline water exist. In this study, they added some baking soda to the water and tested for cholesterol (Reduction in cardiovascular risk by sodium-bicarbonate mineral water in moderately hypercholesterolemic young adults. J Nutr Biochem. 2010 Oct;21(10):948-53). The result was that systolic blood pressure decreased significantly after four weeks of bicarbonate water consumption, without meaningful differentiation between weeks 4 and 8. Then significant reductions in total cholesterol by 6.3%, LDL cholesterol, the bad cholesterol by 10%. The conclusion was that: "Sodium-bicarbonate mineral water improves lipid profile in moderately hypercholesterolemic young men and women and could, therefore, be applied in dietary interventions to reduce cardiovascular risk." This water had no antioxidants in there just baking soda. I think I found the answer in this study (Effect of electrolyzed high-pH alkaline water on blood viscosity in healthy adults Journal of the International Society of Sports Nutrition 2016 13:45) and it was not alkalinity or the minerals in the water. It was viscosity. This was a randomized, double-blind study with one hundred healthy adults. After exercise-induced dehydration participants were randomized to rehydrate with an electrolyzed, high-pH (alkaline) water or standing water. The result was that electrolyzed, high-pH water reduced blood viscosity by an average of 6.30% making it more easy for the blood to flow through the bloodstream compared to 3.36% with standard purified water. What does blood viscosity mean? Viscosity is the internal friction of blood flow. The higher the viscosity, the harder the blood. For example, water has a lower viscosity then honey. Drinking alkaline water can be good only because of the lower viscosity and nothing else. For research into sports drinks and nutrition, this is a topic of great interest.

For general public health as well. Highly viscous blood will have a harder time going thru bloodstream forcing the heart to work harder. Heart will have to have stronger and more powerful contractions to do the extra pumping and in the time that can weaken the heart muscle. Also, viscous blood will raise the blood pressure, and it will be more likely for the blood to form clots inside arteries and veins. If blood is sticky due to dehydration or fat in the bloodstream or other factors, the blood flow is impaired, and the intercellular communication is impaired. The stickier the blood the harder is for the body to undergo cellular detoxification. There is so far a solid understanding, and large number of studies that have been done and showed that elevated blood thickness is associated with heart disease and conditions like lupus and diabetes. Diabetes, smoking, chronic inflammation, also increases the viscosity of blood. Aspirin and warfarin and other blood thinners work by chemically inhibiting blood fragments known as platelets to clump and form clots. That is why an aspirin a day is usually prescribed to a patient who already had a heart attack or has some other sort of cardiovascular problems. Aspirin or warfarin does not, in reality, alter the thickness (viscosity) of blood and hart still need to pump harder and blood pressure are still elevated they just make it harder for blood to form clots. Fluid dynamics is a big science in space agencies and warfare and in general research of propulsion systems. It seems, and this is just consideration that somehow alkaline water has lower viscosity. It acts as a mechanism that will increase the fluidity of the blood and detoxification in the cellular level and increase hydration of the cells and will release the pressure on the cardiovascular system. How does it do it I do not know, and I can only speculate. When insects land on the surface some of them can even walk on water due to the surface tension. When fluidity is increased, the capability for intercellular water chemical interactions increase and body can go into detoxification easier so inflammation will drop.

The new age talks about Hunza water or living water or structured water is just about water fluidity. The more water structures, the more fluidity it will have. An extreme example will be the water that took the shape of crystal and is completely geometrically aligned, i.e. the ice. There is forth aggregate state of water, and many people do not know about this, but yes there is the fourth state of water. The fourth state is the form of state between liquid water and ice, where ice is being the crystal. And that is the state of the liquid crystal when water molecules are in order like in ice but are still in liquid form. You probably heard about LCD monitors. LCD is liquid crystal display. Structured water is structured like a liquid crystal. When water is in this state, it has the highest fluidity off all. Molecules remain mobile but move together. So far it is shown that this water has measurably different characteristics in molecular stability, a negative electrical charge, greater fluidity, molecular alignment, and can also absorb certain spectra of light more efficiently. Some of the water in the healthy human body is already liquid crystalline/structured state. Cell membranes and collagen are also considered to be liquid crystals. There was an experiment in which structure water consumption effected red blood cells in formations known as Rouleaux formation where red blood cells are stacked together in long chains. It happens with increased serum proteins, particularly fibrinogen and globulins and when red blood cells lose their electrical charge. After patient drinks a small amount of structured water, the Rouleaux formation is broken under the microscope and red bool cells have a visible glow or charge around them that repel each other and are swimming in single mode indicating a high zeta potential. Does this have any medical significance I do not know?

There is a supplement on the market that can force the water to arrange itself and it was kind of interesting to me to see what this kind of supplement can do. For example, the average surface tension of water is typically measured in dynes/cm. Ordinary water has a surface tension of 74 dynes, the surface tension of distilled water is 72 dyn/cm, the boiling water is around 58. Hot water has lower surface tension; it is not the temperature that cleans it is lowering of water surface tension that allows hot water to be a better cleanser. Soaps and detergents further lower the surface tension. The structured water has the tension of 48 dyn/cm. There are videos where we can see how to structure water absorbs phytochemicals from tea in comparison to regular with a significant rate of more extraction. When we look at the cellular level, the same thing happens. Structured water increases the rate of flow of both water and oil soluble nutrient across the cell membranes. It is known because of the nuclear magnetic resonance and other techniques that water surrounding our cells is highly structured and organized like liquid crystals especially water around proteins. The only way to create structured water is by special supplements design to do so. Everything else is not scientific, and the results are not supported by science. Vortexing water, music, infrared light, minerals, Earth's Schumann resonance frequencies, crystals all have nothing to do with structuring the water. Structured water is not natural water. There are some more or less structured parts of waters in nature, but rivers and streams and oceans are not structured water.

The only supplement that I know that can do something is Crystal Energy created by "weird" child prodigy new age pentagon employed dr. Patrick Flanagan. He worked for Pentagon, NASA, NSA, CIA, the Office of Naval Research, Tufts University Aberdeen Proving Grounds for the Department of Unconventional Weapons and Warfare and he believes he is the reincarnation of Nicola Tesla and had written the books on sacred geometry and sacred mathematics and other new age stuff. He is unconventional, but his scientific method is sound, so it was kind of off-putting to me to do this research at first. Several scientific papers by Flanagan, about silica hydride, have been published in peer-reviewed journals. Well, Nikola Tesla himself was unconventional too but had singlehandedly invented the 21 century. Dr. Patrick Flanagan got his idea by studying some streams in Himalayas Hunza Valley that had some of the colloidal minerals in water that people drink. These colloidal minerals had an impact on the water and increased its structured form, and that is how he artificially recreated and increased the formula. It was an improved replica of the glacial water. Hunza water has a surface tension value of 58 dynes/cm. Distilled water is not structured water. Only minerals in the water have the potential to force the molecules of H2O to organize. Also, water needs to be pure without a large number of other minerals or chemicals to be able to do it completely. Even filthy water can become more fluid with the addition of this artificially created colloidal mineral but not to the full extent. These colloidal minerals are made out of silica and are artificial. There are 342 natural structures of silica; he made the 343rd structure. The unique form where there are tiny spheres five nanometers in diameter that are so small and have an electric charge of minus 100 millivolts. That is a tenth of the volt in extremely small parts, so it is actually very powerful charge, and when added to the water they attract water molecules and form structures around the colloids, and they all distribute themselves evenly through the liquid. It lowers the surface tension and makes water wetter so things can pass through water more easily and water can pass through things more efficiently too, like going through cell membranes. That will help to hydrate the cells and will increase the rate of transfer of nutrients and waste helping to detoxify the cell. In some studies they calculated to be as much as 2.5 times faster. In fluid dynamics doubling the velocity results in a 64 times increase in the competence. If you double the speed of the river, it can carry 64 times as much material. Structured water, in theory, will increase the speed at which your cells work. It will facilitate the nutrient transfer, water with nutrients coming in through the cell wall and toxins coming out. It will increase the fluidity of the lymphatic system and the circulatory system. How much, in reality, will drinking structured water contribute to overall health and if at all would make any difference I do not know. In cases of dehydration for sure. If we have a hangover or drink a lot of coffee or running the marathon. I will content myself with just clean water and natural foods so far.

Increasing fluidity of blood is not a good idea if we live in nature because of the uncontrollable bleeding. The injuries were a regular part of any animal life. Today maybe not so much but this is still a concern. If you drink structured water and have a car accident, you have a big problem. So far I did not try to drink it, maybe in the future I will give it a try. What Dr. Patrick did after the development of this silica micro clusters were even more interesting to me. He found the way to incorporate the pure hydrogen atom inside the sphere of this artificially created silica thus obtained a system to catch active hydrogen (or negatively ionized hydrogen) inside. Due to the active hydrogen, silica hydride (Megahydrate) is now the most potent antioxidant known to man. So far all scientific studies done have validated the fact that ionized hydrogen is the most potent universal antioxidant ever created. The real problem with most or all of the natural antioxidants is that they became free radicals after giving off their electron and this include vitamin C, vitamin E, etc. That is the reason why when taking antioxidant supplement the overall benefits to the body can be harmful because of the unbalance of our bodies natural defenses. Recycling of the antioxidants is our bodies natural way in which biochemistry functions. Only supplemental antioxidant that can in theory work is just negatively ionized hydrogen that will give its electron and do nothing else except go out of the system. There are some other ways we can force antioxidants in our cells like taking liposomal vitamin C and some other ways. Vitamin C, for example, is a huge molecule that has the sole job to deliver one atom of hydrogen. Just one. When vitamin C gives the electron, it becomes dehydroascorbic acid (DHA) in the body, and that means it has lost its hydrogen. It is now an oxidized form of ascorbic acid (vitamin C) that do not do much except being pro-oxidant itself. All of the antioxidants have different structures and are designed to go to different places in the body, but all of their jobs is to deliver free electron or in other words negatively ionized hydrogen. The vitamin E, vitamin C, and other antioxidants in nature and our body are just a delivery mechanism for hydrogen. Silica hydride byproducts are hydrogen gas and water. And that is it. Silica Hydride is one of the rare antioxidants that do not become a free radical itself after neutralizing other free radicals. There are some others. I will do more analysis of this topic in the chapter about antioxidants in book three of the series. There are a bunch of scientific studies done on this, last time I checked there were 77 of them when I typed silica hydride in PubMed search engine. Here are some of them (Antioxidant Capability and Efficacy of Mega-H™ Silica Hydride, an Antioxidant Dietary Supplement, by In Vitro Cellular Analysis Using Photosensitization and Fluorescence Detection Journal of Medical Food Volume 5, Number 1,2002) (Antioxidant capacity of silica hydride: a combinational photosensitization and fluorescence detection assay. Free Radic Biol Med. 2003 Nov 1;35(9):1129-37.) (Evaluation of Hydroxyl Radical-Scavenging Abilities of Silica Hydride, an Antioxidant Compound, by a Fe21-EDTA-Induced 2-Hydroxyterephthalate Fluorometric Analysis J Med Food 6 (3) 2003, 249–253) (Protective effects of silica hydride against carbon tetrachloride-induced hepatotoxicity in mice. Food Chem Toxicol. 2010 Jun;48(6):1644-53).

Alternatively, there is a simplified method. There is a device that can measure oxidative reduction potential. It is called Oxidative Reduction Potential (ORP) Meter. Oxidation-reduction potential, or ORP, is a measurement that indicates the degree to which a substance is capable of oxidizing or reducing another substance. ORP is an accurate measure of the reducing capacity of antioxidants in a liquid, but it does not necessarily measure effectiveness in scavenging free radicals. The ORP is generally used in conjunction with other methods to give an accurate indication of the possible biological benefits of a compound, but at the end, it can have the possibility to tell us the overall state of the water we want to drink. A positive ORP reading indicates that a substance is an oxidizing agent. If the reading is high, the oxidation is high. For instance, if a substance has ORP reading of +300 mv, it will be three times more oxidizing then the substance that has a reading of +100 mv. Also, it goes in other direction as well. If a substance has negative reading, it will be the reducing agent. Or in other words antioxidant. The lower the reading, the more anti-oxidizing capability of the substance is. For instance, a substance with ORP reading of -300 mv is three times more anti-oxidizing then the substance that has the reading of -100 mv. pH is not deciding factor when it comes to the water. The ORP reading is. It was created for the beer and wine industry. The wine master can put the ORP meter in the barrel, and it will tell him when the fermentation is over. In the pool industry, they put it in the water to measure if the water is oxidizing enough to kill the mold and bacteria so the pool boy will know when to put more chlorine in. Oxidizing kills us too. We do not want to drink something that has positive ORP reading. It will still the electrons from our cells and force them to oxidase and die.

We do not want to speed up oxidation in our bodies, it is already happening naturally, and we are already overfilled with toxins. Fiji is about 350 on ORP, Aquafina 350. Fiji is from pristine spring in Fiji and Aquafina is from Pepsi Colas plants in the US. Tap water has average ORP of +370, Dasani is around 290, Penta water that claims to be energized and ultra-purified through a patented physics process is around 340, SmartWater that people like to drink in the gym is 300, Sprite is around 480, Coke is 410, Gatorade 510, wine 232, Starbucks coffee 175, swimming pools are 475, for water disinfection it is 600, for water sterilization it is 800, distilled water is around 220, alkaline water is the same as distilled, Odwalla Orange Juice 240, Red Bull 460, beer 315, tequila 315, Smirnoff vodka 220. Expensive Essentia Ionized Alkaline 9.5 pH Bottled Water is 179 (it has sodium bicarbonate added, and it is tap water purified through micro-filtration, UV lighting and reverse osmosis; no chlorine or fluoride, and it claims to be enhanced with pure minerals and restructured through ionic separation which by now you know that structuring water in this manner does not work and you can make this at home if you just add baking soda to distilled water and drop of some organic mineral solution supplement). Evamor with a pH of 9,18 and with similar claims like Essentia is 174 on ORP. When you stick ORP meter into the tomato you will probably get something around negative 50 charges if it is still on the vine, in the supermarket, it will be around 170 positive. Best of the green tea will give a reading around 80 probably because of the water they are boiled. Freshly squished juices might go up to minus 100.

We can add Megahydrate to make antioxidant rich structured distilled water and it will drop to minus 500 ORP, but again I personally don't drink structured antioxidant rich water. I get my nutrients from food. It can be beneficial as an added supplement in individuals with high blood pressure. If you have normal blood pressure, then structured water can lower your blood pressure too much and can make your blood prone to excessive bleeding. When this thing first pop out in the supplement industry there where a lot of flak from Harvard scientific medical review and that this is alternative, not a scientific scam and that people should be careful not to trust anything that is not licensed by regular medical institutions and that all of this claims are scientifically impossible. After many of the published scientific studies in peer review journals, flack was gone, but silence emerged. Now it has much more scientific backing, and it is somewhat on the solid ground. Some in vivo studies of the compound showed that it can be gym supplement too and that it has a significant ability to reduce lactic acid build-up in muscles by one-half after exercise and that increases cellular ATP (adenosine triphosphate) production by up to a factor of 4 times, so it is like creatine just better. Also, benefits include the same line of benefits that natural antioxidant does like protection and repair of DNA, neutralization of harmful toxins like fluoride, chlorine, etc., protection against radiation damage, removal of heavy metals from the body and so on. Maybe in the future, I would do some more research into this subject by reviewing more of the studies.

After the clean food and the clean water, there are two more things we need to take into account. The clean air and bad habits. When we talk about the quality of the air, there is nothing much that we can do except move to another place. If you live in cities with air pollution like Beijing, then that is probably a good idea. Air pollution exposure that we know of for the last 30 years of research are connected with respiratory conditions (including asthma and changes in lung function), adverse pregnancy outcomes (such as preterm birth), cardiovascular diseases, adverse effects on children's brain development, increasing overall inflammation in the body and cancer risk and even death. Sometimes the linking air pollution with health problems is visible, as in the Bhopal Disaster. In one more notable incident in 1952, in London, polluted air killed around 4000 people. Because burning of the coal in homes for heating and coal-fired power plants air had become so polluted that literary suffocated people. It was known as the Great Smog. In the US living in the polluted cities was associated with a 16% increase in total mortality rate, 27% with cardiovascular and 28% cancer death rate compared to the non-air polluted cities. It worsens asthma and enhances the risk of developing it at the first place, it overburdens and can trigger liver diseases, increases the risk of diabetes and like any other pollution causes chronic inflammation with damage to DNA and shortens the life.

There is no public safety policy to air pollution except banning lead in gasoline and forcing heavy industry and other heavy air pollutants out of populated areas as much as it can be done. Campaigns to go walking and go with the bicycle to work might be romantic, but there are not practical. Some research that was done on air toxicity estimated that even 10 to 20 percent of overall cancer could be caused by air pollution. However, with air pollution, the effects take a long time to surface, and the direct link is hard to prove. World Health Organization in 2013 finally concluded that outdoor air pollution is a proven carcinogen to humans. If you live in places where air pollution is high it might be a good idea to limit the time of your jogging and exercise outside, stay as far as you can from heavily trafficked roads, and limit the time that children spend outside. If the air quality is terrible, stay inside with windows closed. Indoor air pollution to can be reduced if a building is well-ventilated and cleaned regularly to prevent the buildup of agents like dust and mold. It is a good idea to have high-quality vacuum cleaners and to clean dust and mold regularly.

On top of that if you live in a highly polluted area having an air purifier in the room is also a good idea with a lot of indoor plants. Plants clean air, making them part of what NASA calls nature's life support system. NASA does a lot of this kind of research for purposes of closed indoor colonies on places like Mars. It has been confirmed that adding potted plants to a room reduce the number of air particulates. Plants absorb air, or in other words plans absorb carbon dioxide and release oxygen, but at the same time they filter the air and absorb some of the particulates. Also, microorganisms that are present in the potting soil are also accountable for much of the air cleaning effect. Some plants, in particular, are very good at removing pollutants. A superstar of filtering formaldehyde, for example, is bamboo palm. They are able to grow as much as 12 feet high, making them exciting (and pet-friendly) indoor additions. Because they can be so big is one of the reasons they are able to filter so much of the air. Air purifiers remove almost everything from the air like pollen, air born viruses, dust, odors from cooking and pets, cigarette smoke and so on.

Home perfuming aerosols are toxic also. Plug-in air fresheners produce significant levels of formaldehyde. Burning incense can create inflammation in our lungs because we will breathe in some of the smoke and that smoke will have tiny chemical particles that are toxic and will become trapped in our lungs causing inflammation. The researchers had, for instance, found that some regular chemicals like sandalwood, agarwood are more toxic than tobacco smoke. In 2013, study with 2,000 pregnant women, the International Journal of Public Health reported that air fresheners increase the rate of lung infections in babies dramatically. A 2007 study also found that using air fresheners as little as once a week can raise the risk of asthma in adults. There are more than 100 unknown synthetic chemicals in these fragrances. Glade, for example, keep the list of chemicals as a closely-guarded secret. They do release a master list of nearly 1,500 chemicals that they use in all of their fragranced products because they are required by law, but they do not tell you which chemicals are in which products. When you are breathing in this particles, it is the same as injecting them into the vein. There is no difference if chemical is going to go into the bloodstream thru lungs or thru needle in the vein. Most of these secret chemicals are not scientifically researched, but some of them are like for example volatile organic compounds (VOC) and naphthalene. In studies done on them, both substances caused tissue damage and cancer in the lungs of rats and mice in laboratory studies. Most of the scented candles are made with paraffin and contain VOC. The oil by-product releases ultra-small particles that will contain toxins like benzene, acetone, and toluene. These toxins are carcinogens and are usually seen in diesel emissions. In the study done in the UK that was done on more than 14,000 pregnant women, aerosol sprays were associated with depression in the mothers, headaches and diarrhea and ear infections in their babies. Air pollution is silent but as much toxic input as anything else in this toxic world. World Health Organization (WHO), does reports on air pollution and mortality. In their estimates, air pollution is one of the world's leading killers. Around three million people in the world die each year due to air pollution. In India alone, around half a million people die each year due to air pollution while in the United States, around 41,000 people are estimated to die early because of air pollution. Problem with air pollution is that it is a silent killer. It kills quietly and relentlessly, and the cause is hard to pinpoint. However, air pollution resulting in death is only a minor part of the overall problem that air pollution is causing. Deaths are not the only consequence. There is breathing problems, asthma and bronchitis.

Workers who are constantly exposed to dust particles are known to die from silicosis. Silicosis gives you years of misery before you die.

There is also energy pollution, not just chemical and particle pollution of the air. Man-made sources of EMF radiation such as power lines, mobile phones, computers, Wi-Fi routers, TVs, microwave ovens, radar and radio transmitters provide continuous low-level radiation. It is just one more strain on our own already weakened immune system. Electromagnetic pollution is a by-product of our modern technologically driven environment, and so far there is no reliable option for any form of protection. The situation can only get worse. The environment is already too saturated and overcrowded by the electromagnetic spectrum from all kinds of different technology's used. The International Agency for Research on Cancer (IARC) - the research arm of WHO - classifies extremely low-frequency magnetic fields as Group 2B human carcinogen. What do you think how much of the low electromagnetic wave energy is pulsing right thru you as we speak? Sweden lists electromagnetic fields as class 2 carcinogens. Tobacco is class 2 carcinogen too. That will be all of the cell towers, satellites and other military equipment, the broadcast signals and all of our home appliances. Type 2 carcinogen. The opinions of researchers about the influence of electromagnetic pollution on living organisms are divided. In 20 years from 1980 to 2002 around 200 epidemiological types of research were written regarding the impacts of electromagnetic fields produced by power transmission lines on human beings and what is the conclusion? Well, there isn't one. Someone is trying to hide the truth very efficiently. About 60% of studies done have found no negative correlation and no adverse effects, but 40% reported some smaller or more significant adverse effects caused. Mix results from the studies resulted in fear from lawsuits. Many of the companies themselves have resorted by their own funds to start locating power lines underground, rerouting them and redesigning products (electric appliances and computer monitors) to minimize EMF exposure.

However, again there was corruption involved in the conducting of these studies. In the U.S. most of the studies were funded by big business by themselves meaning electric power generation, transmission, and sales industries and almost all of them found no correlation. Only semi-independent studies were funded in Europe by some governmental agencies and universities, and most of these European studies conclude that long-term exposure to high level of EMF radiation is associated to a broad assortment of health issues and should be avoided. Electromagnetic pollution is so prevalent in our modern world that there are no safe zones from it and there is no solution to it even if proven to be hazardous. The human body is made up of minerals, ions and water and it is just one big antenna. It is a strong conductor of energy, and it picks up energy from the ether. There are molecules in our body that do have an electric charge to them, and that charge is what makes them do their job. Mostly hormones and especially some of the enzymes can be most affected by EMF exposure because they depend on their charge to do their job in the body. Proteins also use the electrostatic interaction between different amino acids to take their exact shape. If EMF exposure is strong enough to disturb even one of these electrostatic interactions in the proteins, the result is a non-functional enzyme/hormone and a disrupted metabolic process. This statement is not just some bro science advice, and it is proven with different types of experiment that strong EMF field do disrupt some hormones and some enzymes that are more prone to it. Strong EMF exposure health result are reduced immune function, increased stress response (hormonal), altered gene expression, disruption in melatonin production (sleep-regulating hormone) and DNA damage. As troubling as these potential health effects are the worst is yet to come.

Our entire brain is nothing more than EMF machine. Different militaries had even studied EMF exposure to the brain for a long time. Different frequency EMF exposure have the potential to affect our nervous system function and that is what worries me the most. This can be turned into some very nasty military applications and technologies with no counterstrategies and with no proof of exposure. Our nervous system is fundamentally an electrical one, so the potential for disruption by EMF's is significant. In some regular circumstances sleep disruption has been correlated with EMF. Some individuals are more hypersensitive to low-frequency EMFs then others. They can experience symptoms like weakened immune system, chronic fatigue with loss of energy inability to concentrate, irritability, headaches and so on. The worst thing of all is that rarely any medical doctor will ever correlate these with EMF radiation exposure sensitivity. Most of MD today think of EMF as heating of the brain problem with our mobile phone kind of a deal. And that is a problem also. Even if you are not hypersensitive and are just regular individual studies showed that this low-level exposure forces the body to produce heat stress proteins in the brain, a form of temporary protective measure that is harmful if this stress response of microwaving our brain is chronic. Electro-proofing your house or reducing your EMF exposure as it fits into your budget as a precaution is a reasonable idea if you live close to the cell towers or other strong EMF fields. Avoiding EMF's is the first step, like putting Wi-Fi out of the bedroom and if you talk on the cell phone for an extended period getting the earplugs is a good idea too.

In nature, we will be running barefoot so any form of EMF will not affect us. Today we wear isolating shoes and can accumulate so much charge. Sometimes usually in winter when the air is dry, we can get static electricity discharge from fingers when we touch something. In the normal condition for any animal that lives on this planet, grounding is a nonstop deal because all animals walk barefoot. Well, all instead of humans. So you need to do a natural thing and ground yourself. Grounding is the process of using direct contact with the earth to disperse any electromagnetic pollution that had accumulated in your body. Just one touch in one millisecond will discharge you of all static electricity that you have accumulated. When you walk barefoot like any other animal, you absorb all of the free electrons from the Earth into your body that spread throughout your tissues. The procedure of touching the earth is sufficient to preserve your body at the same negatively-charged electrical potential that the Earth as a planet itself has. You can try to ground some of the stuff in your home like mats for example. Will this have any benefit on your health, I do not know. There is no consensus in the scientific field. It could stop the adverse effects of EMF it there are any.

Constant state of our body positive static charge in our modern environment is real, and you can test this on yourself. The only question is, does this unnatural charge doing us any real harm? With conflicting studies, it might be a good idea to protect yourself "just in case". Lead in the paint, for example, was considered safe in the past and there was no problem with asbestos too. Lead paint was seductive to children. The greatest danger was for small children who can put lead or lick lead painted objects because they tasted sweet. I have issues with trusting anything that government or industry says. From lead gasoline particles in the air (lead gasoline is still used in some countries in the world) to EMF in the air to the ELF in the air to the stratospheric aerosol particles in the air. External extremely low-frequency (ELF) electromagnetic fields induce electric fields and currents inside the body which can that cause the nerve and muscle stimulation and changes in nerve cell excitability in the central nervous system. In non-scientific terms, extremely low EMF frequencies had the potential to resonate with a human brain if they have the same frequency in which our brain operates and that is not nice "Hollywood style" telepathy. It is, and I will say it in this way "problematic" because there where development programs in the Soviet Union and the US as well for the use of this kind of resonance technology in military applications. Was this kind of military program development successful I do not know. Even if not weaponized, sometimes we can find unexpected correlations. As an example, most breast tumors become resistant to tamoxifen (Nolvadex), and it has been shown that ELF-EMF reduces the efficacy of tamoxifen in a manner similar to tamoxifen resistance. By exposing breast cancer cells in line MCF-7 to ELF-EMF fields, these ELF-EMF will alter the expression of estrogen receptor cofactors, which will then result in tamoxifen resistance in vivo. The problem is that much of this science has military applications. I cannot do an objective review of ELF-EMF influence on the human condition. I do not know what the truth is. Tease technologies are under the stamp of classified information. If you want, then do more research yourself. My suggestion is that you do not self-experiment with God Helmet and similar devices that can be found on the market and wrapping your head in tinfoil just looks silly and doesn't even work.

Maybe we cannot influence toxic level in our air or radiation, but we could try to do the thing that is in our power like getting rid of bad habits. When we talk about healthy lifestyle people immediately start to think about their bad habits like smoking and drinking alcohol. However, what about other bad habits like drinking coffee and eating meat. Do we think that eating meat is health promoting and normal? Maybe we just need to remember the fact that it took more than 7000 studies and more than half of century of arguing back and forth with scientific community and industry until the first Surgeon General report versus smoking was eventually published and many more years after until it was finally acknowledged that inhaling smoke might be a bad idea. Inhaling smoke back in the 50s was considered good, and all of the physicians smoked. The physician lounges had air that you could cut with a knife. Hospitalized patients were free to smoke too, in bed even, so long as open oxygen was not flowing. Do we think that physicians now are going to know or tell us the truth about anything else? There are no nutritional exams in college, and I will add intentionally by design from the industry. They want the doctors to do their job and make big pharma money and keep people sick and docile. If you wait for your regular medical doctor to give you real advice you are going to wait for another 50 years at least or more. I will skip the broad analysis of the adverse effects of smoking and drug abuse because it is not much about that topic that isn't already acknowledged. Smoking is so bad that for example after quitting there is still elevated level in C reactive protein (inflammation marker) in the body that remained significantly higher up to 5 years following cessation.

Furthermore, C reactive protein levels were reduced to be equal to the normal levels detected in people who never smoked only in individuals who had quit for over 20 years. Similarly, if you think drinking alcohol is just correlated with car crashes and liver disease you are seriously wrong. Consumption of alcohol in hundreds of different studies that had been done linked it to more than 60 diseases. People who drink on a regular basis will have many different health implications. Their habit is going to affect not just the health status of their liver but almost every organ in their bodies.

The developing fetal brain and adolescent brain also are primarily vulnerable to the toxic effects of alcohol. If mother drinks during pregnancy that will have an adverse effect on fetal brain development. Alcohol restricts to some extent the production of vasopressin (ADH). It is a hormone produced in the hypothalamus and are secreted from the posterior pituitary gland. Dehydration after alcohol consumption is a consequence of this restriction. People who regularly drink more than one standard drink per day are at higher risk of long-term health conditions. Even if you do not feel the effect of the drink, you did yourself harm. And that is not all. Alcohol consumption releases excess GABA and dopamine. If too much of these neurotransmitters get released situation can change dramatically from feeling nice and relaxed to increased heart rate, shortness of breath, increased levels of both aggression and depression, high blood pressure, delusions, hallucinations, night terrors, spasms, and so on. Excess drinking causes the liver to accumulate fat, which can lead to fatty liver disease especially if you are already obese. Even one drink a day may increase the person's risk for breast cancer by 4% because alcohol has a pro-estrogenic influence on the cells. Cancers that are responsive to hormones will also have positive respond to substances that influence hormones like for instance breast cancer. The increase of the order of 4% is done just by one small alcoholic drink/day. If you drink three or more drinks a day, then your breast cancer risk goes up by, imagine this 40-50 percent. Around 5 percent of all breast cancers in the US are attributed just to alcohol consumption and around 1 to 2 percent to light drink alone. Combine this with pro-estrogenic effects of POPs and plastic and all other xenoestrogens. Besides breast cancer, 3.6% of other types of cancers are caused directly by chronic alcohol drinking, and these include the liver, the colorectum and those of the upper digestive tract ones. The International Agency for Research on Cancer (IARC) official UN body under WHO considers ethanol as a carcinogen to humans (Group 1). Beside ethanol alcoholic beverages are multicomponent mixtures that can be containing several different carcinogenic compounds, such acetaldehyde, aflatoxins, and ethyl carbamate. Ethanol is considered the most important carcinogen in alcoholic beverages, but there are other carcinogenic compounds as well.

The biological mechanisms by which alcohol intake increases the risk of cancer are not fully understood, but the primary mechanisms are likely to include a genotoxic effect of acetaldehyde, the induction of cytochrome P450 2E1 and associated oxidative stress, increased estrogen concentration, a role as a solvent for tobacco carcinogens, changes in folate metabolism, and changes in DNA repair. For cancers of the digestive tract, especially those of the upper digestive tract, acetaldehyde (derivate from alcohol that creates itself almost instantly when you sip on an alcoholic beverage) has been highlighted as a likely and important causal pathway. That metabolite is so toxic it is terrible. For colorectal cancer, in addition to the genotoxic effect of acetaldehyde, there may be the involvement of folate: alcohol may act through folate metabolism or synergistically with low folate intake. Bacteria in our mouths oxidase ethanol into acetaldehyde almost instantaneously. Even a single sip is enough to cause high concentrations of acetaldehyde even without drinking, there is still effect for example if you use alcoholic mouthwash. In this study (A single sip of a strong alcoholic beverage causes exposure to carcinogenic concentrations of acetaldehyde in the oral cavity. Food Chem Toxicol. 2011 Sep;49(9):2103-6) they found that holding single sip of a strong alcoholic beverage for 5 seconds in the mouth and then spitting it out formed carcinogenic concentrations of acetaldehyde in the oral cavity instantly and the exposure continued for at least 10 min. So even washing your mouth with it is cancer promoting. There is also more to booze then just cancer. Alcohol rises lipids in the blood and also blood pressure. That will increase the risk of raised cholesterol, hypertension, stroke and heart attack. It causes cardiomyopathy, myocarditis and it also causes arrhythmia.

However, wait red wine has long been considered the elixir of heart health. We can all remember the scam named French paradox. French paradox was love affair of everyone. In 1980 some French scientist tried to explain the correlation between high fat intake, and especially saturated one from lots of meat and dairy products with lower heart attack rate in France especially when compared with one in Britain for example. It was statistical proof that cholesterol and all of meat and eggs and cheese do not cause heart disease and even if they do we can just add some nice red wine after the meal and what more do you want. Red wine is some kind of superfood. However, correlation is not causation, and one factor that had been ignored was, and I will write it again was, the past tense, that the French diet was generally healthier than other nations at the time. They had been eating four times more vegetables then counterpart countries and it was a form of a semi Mediterranean diet. However, it turned out to be no paradox at all. It turned out that French physicians underreport heart disease on death certificates as much as 20% according to WHO. If we correct that statistical error, then no benefit of wine. The only good thing in wine are phytochemicals from grapes so if you want these, the better option will be just regular grape juice and the even better option will be to eat fresh grapes. Some other studies support alcohol and heart disease connection. Low levels of alcohol consumption can raise levels of high-density lipoprotein (good cholesterol), HDL. So they had the idea that moderate drinking protects against cardiovascular disease by raising HDL, which would make sense biologically if you already have razed levels of cholesterol. They need this kind of studies to calm people down from time to time. Alternatively, we will stop eating animal products if we fear cholesterol. Also, some small amount of alcohol consumption like a glass of wine a day had been found to have beneficial changes in factors that influence blood clotting, and that will mean fewer chances for thrombosis of any sort like blood clots in the brain, block arteries in the heart and so on. Blood clots are the most common kind of stroke. Booze is what chemists call amphiphilic. It interacts favorably with both polar and non-polar molecules same as any other amphiphilic substance like soaps and detergents. So if you add rubbing alcohol to grease, the alcohol starts mixing with it. It blends in by going in between the long fatty chains. It does the same thing in the bloodstream.

Alternatively, you can take aspirin; it has a similar effect to blood clots without liver damage and cancer. We do not need alcohol for this. What about coffee? Do we think caffeine is something good for our brain or bad or neutral? So far research has no evidence to associate link between coffee and an increased risk of heart disease or cancer. Some of the studies found decreased overall mortality by the same small amount, and some other found that it does the opposite. If we take an average conclusion from them, it will be approximately very small or no significant effect on longevity. What coffee seems to increase is cognitive function and reduce the risk of depression. So did we found our amphetamine drug free of charge? Coffee's does have a high concentration of antioxidants providing cells protection from oxidative stress and inflammation. It is the bean after all. However, we can get other nontoxic beans to get all of the benefits that coffee bean has, and we should not confuse the benefits of coffee as unique. Most of the antioxidant rich foods will have the same effect. When people talk about the benefit of coffee, they tell half-truth when insinuating that it is the benefit of that bean only and that we would not have the similar benefits if we eat another type of beans. For example, cocoa beans have caffeine too but much more of the beneficial polyphenol antioxidants and much more health benefits so talking about the benefit of coffee is little misleading.

To get to the truth, we should look into studies of pure caffeine and its effect on the body because that is the reason people drink coffee in the first place. We could get most of the benefits of coffee with decaf too. It is caffeine that we need to investigate and not just using misleading science to justify our habit. It is the same story as alcohol, finding some benefit that we can also find in other food items without any unique special ability to just coffee bean so that we can justify our caffeine high. So what does the actual caffeine do? We can take it in pills for example or in energy drinks. If we look at the chemical structure of caffeine, we will see that it is very similar to adenosine. Adenosine is chemical in the brain that makes us sleepy. Whenever we are awake adenosine slowly accumulates in our brain. Adenosine binds to the receptors and in time slows our brain activity down. The longer we are awake, the more adenosine accumulate, the more tired we feel. At some point, we will go to sleep. While sleeping concentration of adenosine decline and at morning cycle begins again. Because caffeine is similar to adenosine and acts as adenosine receptor blocker in the brain, it will cancel natural brain chemistry making us feel more alert. For the individuals that regularly drink coffee in extensive amounts, our brains adjust by developing more adenosine receptors, so it takes more caffeine to elicit the same response. Having more adenosine receptors also means more adenosine makes its way into our brains so if we do not drink coffee, we will be more tired than in our regular normal state. In the morning, we will not be fully alert and during the day we will feel more tired if we did not drink our cup that day. It has a half-life of 6 hours meaning half of it will be gone in 6 hours so after 6 hours you will be feeling half of the effect. Couple hours later it will be mostly gone, and we will need another cup. Caffeine also stimulates the body to produce much more adrenaline than needed and that will end up with increased heart rate and anxiety. Caffeine puts the body in a stressful state of fight and flight response leading to increase in anxiety. People who are already overstressed and prone to panic attacks and other pro anxiety conditions can have severe reactions with a tremor in hands and cold sweats and heart palpitations from caffeine. Caffeine also prevents dopamine from getting reabsorbed acting like cocaine in some sense leading to good feeling so by now we are in addictive behavior and have withdrawal symptoms. This dopamine effect is what makes coffee so addictive. The reason why Coca Cola puts caffeine in Coke is precisely because of this. The lethal dose of caffeine is 150mg per kg of the body mass. For a 70kg human, it is 14000mg caffeine. A cup of coffee on average have 150mg. This is not enough to kill but there is still one more fact that people tend to know little about. However, is the one effect that is most important of them all. Adenosine also controls blood flow through the brain.

Caffeine produces cerebral vasoconstriction by antagonizing adenosine receptors. Caffeine-induced cerebral vasoconstriction is well documented

(Separating neural and vascular effects of caffeine using simultaneous EEG-FMRI: differential effects of caffeine on cognitive and sensorimotor brain responses. Neuroimage. 2012 Aug 1;62(1):239-49). 250 mg of caffeine was found to be associated with significant reductions in cerebral perfusion thirty and ninety minutes later around. The value of decreased blood flow in the brain goes from 20% for one small cup of coffee to 40% for 2 or 3 cups. Chronic caffeine use results in an adaptation of the vascular adenosine receptor system presumably to compensate for the vasoconstrictive effects of caffeine. This entire adrenaline bump and stress in the form of I am suffocating and dying, help me, I am your brain without the oxygen is what actually wakes you up because you are about to die literally. That is what your alert state is. Fight or flight stress response. And that is the real job of caffeine, to be one more neurotoxic chemical for defense against pests. If you drink coffee every day, the brain adapts and tries to compensate.

Nevertheless, there is a deadline to what the brain can compensate. The limit is around 400 mg of caffeine a day. Drinking more than that will have vasoconstrictive effects even in the people who are chronic caffeine addicts. What happens is that in expectation of one more coffee cup the brain is going to raise its internal brain pressure. So when we drink coffee, the pressure will drop from vasoconstrictive effects and became normal. If you skip that cup in the morning and skip again in the afternoon the buildup of the internal brain pressure is going to give you a migraine headache. That is the reason why people who are trying to quit usually suffer from headaches that can last for days before brains starts to adapt again to new normalized conditions.

There is more. Caffeine is also frequently utilized as a pre-workout supplement, but caffeine may adversely affect and limit bloodstream flow to heart muscle throughout exercise (Caffeine impairs myocardial blood flow response to physical exercise in patients with coronary artery disease as well as in age-matched controls PLoS One. 2009 May 22;4(5):e566). When we do a physical exercise blood flow has to increase in order to match the increased need for oxygen and caffeine may adversely affect this mechanism too and not just blood supply to the brain. It restricts the blood flow in the heart muscle, but interestingly enough it did not affect blood flow while the study subjects were at rest. When the subjects took caffeine tablets and exercised the blood flow were significantly lower than normal. Blood flow should increase when people exercise do to the more significant demand for energy, but caffeine blocks receptors for adenosine in the heart muscle and blocks specific receptors in the walls of blood vessels. I would not recommend that anyone take caffeine as a pre-workout supplement or for any athlete to drink caffeine before sports. In upper mentioned study after oral administration of caffeine 200 mg bicycle exercise-induced myocardial blood flow decreased by 11% in regular individuals. In subjects who have coronary artery disease decrease was 18% and by 25% in stenotic subjects (with cholesterol deposit narrowing of coronary arteries).

Caffeine is a pesticide that kills insects and other plants. Neurotoxic poison. It has a purpose of defending the coffee plant.

The coffee plant is one of the rare plants in nature that commits suicide. The leaves and beans that fall from the coffee tree have caffeine, and they start to poison the ground. At first, they kill everything that lives in topsoil but as time passes and more and more leaves fall, and more concentration of caffeine in soil rises the more of the root system of the coffee plant itself get affected. Investigations regarding the use of caffeine on plants demonstrated that when the concentration of caffeine gets high enough it begins to distort plant cells and if it gets even higher the result is the death of the plant. People usually try to drink coffee when they are already stressed enough. They have a lot of work, or they need to study for the exam so that constant stressful response full of adrenalin and cortisol up and downs is going to give them adrenal fatigue and overall stressful condition. Adrenal fatigue is not a real disease just made up term. It is not an accepted medical diagnosis. There is a real medical condition called Addison disease which causes adrenal insufficiency. Adrenal fatigue does not cause inadequate production of one or more of these hormones as a result of an underlying disease. Adrenal fatigue is a light form of adrenal insufficiency caused by chronic stress with rapid hormonal ups and downs during the day. It is not as much as insufficiency of the adrenal glands as it is overall fatigue state caused by constant hormonal fluctuations. Trying to take valium to relax or because you are unable to sleep is just going to make things worse. How many people are complaining on their stressful lives? The valid question should be how many of them are caffeine addicts? Keep that in mind the next time you are eyeing that 2nd (or 10th) cup of joe.

After all of this, there is still one more route where toxins can enter our bodies. It is not from food, water, air or radiation. It is through our skin. All cosmetics that we put on our skin penetrate it, get absorbed to our tissue and blood system and then enter our bodies directly. It is worse than eating it because in our digestive system there are acids in the stomach and billions of protective probiotic microorganisms that can help us to some extent. Putting something to our skin is the same as inhaling it or shooting it directly to our vein. If you do not want to eat it, then don't put it on your skin. If you are a woman and you need to dye your hair, then first put some of that ammonia dye into your mouth because that is precisely what you do when you put dye on your head. Many studies had been done on the possible link between hair dye use and cancer for many years, especially link with bladder cancer, leukemia, and lymphomas. Early hair dyes contained some aromatic amines, which were found in the late 1970s to cause cancer in lab animals. Today IARC has established that workplace exposure as a hairdresser or barber is probably carcinogenic to humans. What we know is toxic and also found in most of the hair dyes is formaldehyde (cancer and fetal damage in utero), p-Phenylenediamine (kidney problems and bladder cancer, PPD, in short, is applied as a dye for dark tone colors and is manufactured from coal tar), DMDM hydantoin (immunotoxin, banned for use in Japanese cosmetics), ammonia (respiratory problems and asthma), resorcinol (increase in circulating testosterone levels) , eugenol (cancer, allergies, immune and neurological system toxicity), parabens, lead acetate (for the dark shade, anemia, neurological problems). There is also a list of more than 20 different hair dye chemicals banned by the European Commission so far. Again if you do not want to eat it do not put in on your skin. It will add to overall toxic exposure even if they are not cancerogenic chemicals. Organic hair salons are popping up like mushrooms these days due to the growing toxic awareness.

What about the rest of the cosmetics? In 2017 cosmetics industry on a global scale reached $265 billion in revenue. For products that are used on a daily basis, small effects cumulating over time within large populations can be almost impossible to predict without comprehensive analysis and studies, and that is something nobody wants to invest into. There are some studies that have been done, but that is not an adequate amount. Currently, cosmetic manufacturers have no legal obligation to report health problems from their products.

An excellent example of this is Johnson & Johnson company that has suffered lines of costly court defeats over cases of its talcum powder inducing cancer. And many more cases are still looming. What happened was that internal memos showed that Johnson & Johnson knew about the cancer risk but still decided to misinform and represent talcum powder as an absolutely safe product. So far jury has awarded more than 300 million dollars in damages with hundreds of more lawsuits pending. Memos revealed that decades ago their own employed toxicologists where warning the company that there is a statistically significant association between hygienic talk use and ovarian cancer. It took years but in time there were nine studies done and published in the open literature. They also warned Johnson & Johnson that if they deny this risk, the talk industry will be seen in the public eye as same as the cigarette industry. The main argument of the victim families was that the company knew but deliberately did not present an adequate warning to customers of the risks of using the talk powder in question. The main cancerogenic substance in question was talk that can be found in many everyday household products such as body powders, cosmetics or products designed especially for babies. The International Agency for Research on Cancer lists the perineal use of talc-containing products as possibly carcinogenic to humans. Talc, a naturally occurring mineral, can also sometimes contain a trace amount of asbestos but asbestos is cut from powders back in the 70s and it is not the culprit here, the talk is. It might be safe in the area of sweating armpit, but woman traditionally put the stuff on their genitalia and the genitalia of babies too. Inhaling is also carcinogenic, and people who work with talk are at higher risk. It also raises the risk for fibroid tumors. This kind of tumors has no threat of malignancy. They are composed of muscle cells that overgrow to form a mass or knot within the uterus that is causing swelling, increased urination, and abdominal pain. By age 50 more than 80% of black woman and 70% of white woman have it.

Now we cannot live the life of paranoia and deprivation in fear of every product that is out there. All I can say welcome to the real world of "being informed." Sometimes having high IQ is not very romantic. Stupidity and ignorance might be the bliss down the line. Currently, there are more than 80,000 ingredients used in cosmetic. More than 10,000 of them are industrial chemicals used as cosmetic ingredients. Some of them are reproductive toxins, known carcinogens, and endocrine disruptors. Parabens are preservative used in cosmetics with 75 to 90 percent of cosmetics containing them. Also, parabens are used as fragrance ingredients, but consumers will not find that listed on the label because fragrance recipes are considered trade secrets. What they do is mimic estrogen. They are one of the well-known xenoestrogens. Studies show that methylparaben used on the surface of the skin responds with UVB spectrum of light increasing skin damage, causing aging and DNA damage. They can be present naturally in certain foods but are metabolized when eaten. When applied to the skin they will be absorbed into the body directly to the bloodstream. Going into details about all of these chemicals is useless. Without governmental regulation, you as a consumer cannot read and understand all of the weird chemicals if they are even listed. There are a bunch of them that are known to be toxic. I will just name them and won't go into details just so that we can have some objective view.

DEA (diethanolamine) and DEA compounds (used to make cosmetics creamy, cause liver cancers and cancerous changes in skin and thyroid), dibutyl phthalate or DBP (nail products and some hair sprays, toxic to reproduction and hormone balance), BHA (butylated hydroxyanisole) and BHT (butylated hydroxytoluene) (in moisturizer, makeup, cause cancer and interfere with hormone function), formaldehyde (listed on the label as DMDM HYDANTOIN, DIAZOLIDINYL UREA, IMIDAZOLIDINYL UREA, METHENAMINE, or QUARTERNIUM-15) , synthetic fragrances and parfum (allergies and asthma, cancer and neurotoxicity), PEGs (cancer, used in, moisturizers, conditioners, deodorants), mineral oil (makeup, lotions, in baby oil, soap can have PAHs that cause cancer, are toxic to liver), siloxanes (hair products, moisturizer, makeup, damage the liver and disrupt hormones), sodium lauryl sulfate (SLS) and sodium laureth sulfate (SLES)(shampoo, cleansers, bubble bath, can be contaminated with 1,4-dioxane), triclosan (in anti-bacterial products and sanitizers, interfere with hormone function), chemical sunscreens (inflammation, dermalogical effects, allergic reactions and photogenotoxic (DNA altering) effects and actually promote cancer), aluminum (brain disorders, breast cancer, pro estrogenic effect).

The common woman uses 12 personal care products daily and man about 6 with each product containing a large list of chemicals. Less than 20% of these chemicals are tested for safety by industries safety panels. The just dump them to products literally. They do not have a legal obligation to test them. It would be too expensive for the industry to do double-blind clinical trials for every chemical they put in cosmetics and there are no legal obligations for them to do so. Thus we do not know what these chemicals can do. On cosmetics labels, words like "natural", "herbal", "organic" has no legal definition. That means companies can put chemicals form laboratory and called them natural because they smell like flowers. Herbal Essences from Procter and Gamble, number two shampoo in the US, for example, have the "essences" made from oil, and you will read this as a fragrance on the label. They add a touch of real oils from plants so that they can have a nice picture on the front and misguide you. This real natural essential oil is not what gives them a refreshing smell. Also, citric acid, a natural ingredient that is often found in citrus fruits such as oranges and lemons is there to balance the pH of the shampoo to about 5.5. Shampoos, including brand like Herbal Essences, are kept at a slightly acidic pH level. Citric acid acts as a preservative, and acidic levels are kept because hair appears shinier and lies smoother. Sodium citrate, which is also an Herbal Essences ingredient, achieves the same result as citric acid and is cheaper but they add citric acid beside it. They do that to fool you because if you think that you are smart and know what and from where citric acid is you will think that it must be "natural" shampoo. The worst from all cosmetics on the market are skin whitening creams. They are super toxic. When for example Estee Lauder offers you a chance to help fight breast cancer they are at the same time using chemicals that are linked to cancer. Pink ribbon is so "empowering" to the woman cause. They all know how much real intelligence average woman has.

The way they get away with this is marketing and when somebody asks them why are they using these chemicals they have a defense that these chemicals are a necessity. Without them, there will not be most of the products on shelves because there isn't any other way for manufacturing them. These products will be overly expensive, and most woman will have no money to buy them, and that doses used are so small that they will have no impact on the health of the users. And yes, they know all of this even if there are no clinical trials for most of the chemicals they are using. Some of the workers get dosed all they long. Even now when there are studies that link many of these substances to diseases, there are no laws to force the industry to get rid of them. The FDA does not assess the safety of personal care products. Since 1938 they banned 8 out of more than 12000 chemicals used in cosmetics. They do not even require for all of the ingredients to be listed on the label. Cosmetic companies are self-policing, and compliance with recommendations is voluntary.

After all of this toxicity when people talk of cleansing protocols somehow it turns into esoteric pseudoscience. It is true that most of the detox diets out there are not scientifically proven. It is also the truth that most of the natural traditional detoxifying herbs are also not scientifically proven. However, again some of them have been around for thousands of years of traditional use.

In the end, the best detox is to stop absorbing toxins in the first place. There are programs of dieting that are designed to help reduce inflammation and overall body toxicity that are backed by science. You already know by now what they are. They are natural (meaning in line with human evolution) whole food plant-based diet with a low level of environmental toxin exposure. That is it. If you think that you can eat most of the time anything that you want and go on some cleansing diet for a month or two, in reality, this will have no long-lasting effects. We can find this line of thinking in Traditional Chinese Medicine for example, or in the tradition of Nativity Fast and The Great Fast or Lent practiced by the Eastern Orthodox Churches where only fish is allowed from all animal products, and "real" fast is even without the fish too. However, that will work no more. Most of the babies are born these days already with massive toxic build up. Most of the children in western countries have a visible arteriosclerotic plaque by the age of 7, and a significant portion of them are obese. If we do not regulate our diet on the scientific bases meaning eat the food that science and evolution have defined not our emotional desire, any cleansing protocol is just wasting of time.

There are some scientifically backed methods to lower the toxicity. One of them will be to eat a lot of fiber. Fiber bound to excess of estrogen in the body and can have protective effects against hormonal cancers like breast cancer. Because of all of the xenoestrogens eating an adequate amount of fiber is the right decision. Also, all fat-soluble molecules like cholesterol can only be detoxified by pushing them directly into the digestive tract in the hope that they will bound with fiber and leave the body by excrement and not by kidneys that can only detoxify water-soluble chemicals. Fiber intake is associated with a low level of lead, cadmium, mercury and other heavy metals in the body too. Fiber bound itself to the lead and other heavy metals in such a strong way that makes absorption impossible. Absorption happens later when probiotic bacteria dissolve some of the fiber, so it is not a fail-safe solution. However, in the end, heavy metal bioavailability from animal-based foods was higher than that from vegetable-based foods because of all of fiber and phytochemicals (Cadmium bioavailability from vegetable and animal-based foods assessed with in vitro digestion/caco-2 cell model. J Med Assoc Thai. 2011 Feb;94(2):164-71). In this study just adding kale to the pig kidneys (one of the most abundant sources of cadmium), the toxic exposure was significantly lower. When scientist measure trace element concentrations meaning exposure to lead and cadmium in subjects who changed from a mixed diet to a lactovegetarian diet same things happen (Trace element status in healthy subjects switching from a mixed to a lactovegetarian diet for 12 mo. Am J Clin Nutr. 1992 Apr;55(4):885-90). The plasma and hair concentrations of selenium, copper, and zinc had decreased but those of magnesium had increased. Concentrations of cadmium, lead, mercury in hair was lower. The tendency was towards the increased elimination of lead and cadmium and mercury following the change to the vegetarian diet. Within three months the levels significantly dropped and stay down for the rest of the year following experiment. After switching back to the regular diet, they come back three years later, and levels were back up to the old high values. The story of why selenium decreased by 40% in this study is because European soil (this study was done in Sweden) is severely selenium deficient. Mercury was down 20%, cadmium and lead 50%.

There are scientifically proven specific plant species that can aid in detoxification of heavy metals and other toxins as well because of their high antioxidant potential. Curcumin, for example, became one of the healthiest and most researched plants in the last decades or so. Curcumin reduces the toxicity induced by mercury, chromium, cadmium, arsenic, copper, lead, maintains the liver antioxidant enzyme status and, prevents histological injury, lipid peroxidation, and glutathione (GSH) depletion, and protects against mitochondrial dysfunction. Curcumin has scavenging and chelating properties that can chelate or bound to heavy metals allowing them to be exerted out (Curcumin derivatives as metal-chelating agents with potential multifunctional activity for pharmaceutical applications. J Inorg Biochem. 2014 Oct;139:38-48). We do not need to take a curcumin supplement if we don't have kidney stones; we can just eat cheap turmeric powder mixed with ground pepper (I will explain this in more detail in one of the later chapters). Particular types of fiber and carbohydrates found in seaweed also are able to stick to heavy metals and help them be released out from the body. Seaweed compounds have been found to chelate (stick to and bind) different heavy metals including radioactive strontium (cancer-causing compound) from the body (Alginate enhances excretion and reduces absorption of strontium and cesium in rats. Biol Pharm Bull. 2013;36(3):485-91). Cilantro is also very well-known and a great binder of heavy metals. The preventive effect of Coriandrum sativum, (Chinese parsley) on lead deposition was investigated in a couple of different studies (Preventive effect of Coriandrum sativum (Chinese parsley) on localized lead deposition in ICR mice. J Ethnopharmacol. 2001 Oct;77(2-3):203-8). Administration of Chinese parsley to mice significantly decreased lead deposition in the femur and severe lead-induced injury in the kidneys suggesting that it has chelation affinities tours lead by some undiscovered substance contained in Chinese parsley. Beside this, we have one of the folk remedies for all illnesses in natural medicine, the garlic. When garlic is cut, crushed or chewed, an enzyme called alliinase converts allin to allicin. Allicin in garlic is the actual active compound. It is designed to defend the plant from insects chewing on it. It is responsible for the intense odor of fresh garlic. The way we prepare garlic influences the number of beneficial compounds we receive from it. Because it is not thermostable and only gets created when cells in garlic are damaged, it must be first crushed and left alone for some time and only when eaten raw, only then it will have its germicidal effect. What was interesting is that with antiviral and antimicrobial properties of garlic it is also strong heavy metal detoxifier and no garlic does not have an antiplatelet activity like aspirin. The aim of this Iranian study (Comparison of therapeutic effects of garlic and d-Penicillamine in patients with chronic occupational lead poisoning. Basic Clin Pharmacol Toxicol. 2012 May;110(5):476-81) was to investigate therapeutic effects of garlic and compare it with d-penicillamine (the pharmaceutical grade chelation therapy drug) in patients with chronic lead poisoning. They gave each subject garlic tablet containing 400 mg dried powder garlic that is equivalent to 1200 μg allicin or 2 g fresh garlic. Yes, 2 g of fresh garlic. In this case not raw garlic just regular tablet supplement that you can buy in a store. The supplement will not give you bad breath. Garlic and the pharmaceutical grade drug both reduced lead levels by 20% and the garlic had no side effects. On another hand, there are serious side effects of d-penicillamine. Allicin is known a chelating agent in the treatment of lead poisoning but also that S-allyl cysteine and S-allyl mercaptocysteine, both substances founded in garlic extract, inhibit lead absorption directly from the gastrointestinal tract. In addition, garlic had more clinical improvement than d-penicillamine in a number of clinical manifestations including irritability, systolic blood pressure, headache, decreased deep tendon reflex. The reason for this is that chelation drugs can only reduce the blood levels. The problem is that the heavy metals are not just in the blood but are in the cells and body own mechanism must remove them from the cells where chelation drugs have no impact. However, it looks like that garlic did it just by itself. It helped the entire body not just blood to detoxify. Detoxifying just by drinking water is not a whole solution.

Fat in our body acts like deposit for these toxins. When we start to lose weight toxins get released into the bloodstream. If we are on a diet, it is not enough to go water fasting or juice fasting to detoxify. We need to eat fiber too. We need a lot of healthy bacteria in our intestines to protect us from food toxins and release chemicals that our body need, and we will only get them from fiber-rich food. Another scientifically backed method is to eat antioxidants to neutralize the significant amount of these toxins from doing damage to our DNA. We need antioxidant and fiber-rich toxin free meals so in other word broccoli, carrots, kale, apples, and other vegetables and fruits. That is a healthy diet detoxification plan. Coffee enemas not so much. A large amount of fiber in diet will clean our intestines and feed our probiotic bacteria at the same time. If we want, we can add activated charcoal to the mix to clean our intestines from the inside. What activated charcoal does is it allows harmful drugs and toxins that are in the gut to bind to it. Its permeable surface has a negative electric charge. That is like an antioxidant just it is not, it does not neutralize anything it just binds to it and gets it out. It attracts positively charged ions and gas, and all oxidants and toxins are bound until you poop. This is the reason activated charcoal is often used among patients who suffered from a drug overdose or poisoning since it assists the body in eliminating these unwanted materials by attaching and not allowing them to go free and enter the bloodstream. It is a common ingredient in water filter systems as well because it can trap pesticides, solvents, industrial waste, chemicals, and other impurities.

Besides fiber, we need a large number of antioxidants to protect our cells from toxic damage. Only on top of that, we can try to do common known detoxifying methods like drinking lot of herbal teas and distilled water and green and other vegetable juices, but again we should do that every day just by part of our regular lifestyle and diet. We can only live healthy and help our body do the job. Anything else like detoxifying from time to time will lead to disease. Some scientifically proven chemicals can help our liver do a better job at detoxifying. The liver is the most crucial organ in detoxification beside the kidneys and then the intestinal tract, from the mouth to the colon. Intestinal tract does not only have the task of digestion but also of the elimination of toxins and the prevention of toxins from food to enter the blood at the first stage. Lungs, and bronchi also remove toxins in the form of carbonic gas. If the liver, lungs, and kidneys do not detoxify efficiently, the body needs help from the skin that removes toxins in the form of crystals. Crystals are the remains of the breakdown metabolism of food rich in protein, such as eggs, fish, meat, and dairy. Urea is part of the group of crystals. If you have a strong odor, it might even have clinical significance. If insulin level drops, the body begins to break down fat for fuel, which leads to a buildup of ketones. That accumulation, in turn, may produce a change in body odor, and it might be a sign it is time to see a doctor. If you want to do a trendy keto diet full of protein and low in carbs, you need to know that you are going to have change in body odor and also an impact to the smell of your breath. However, skin is not the primary detoxifying engine in the body. Liver is. If the liver is unable to detoxify for example in cases like cirrhosis, we die. If our kidneys are not able to detoxify we die or use modern technology to prolong our life like dialysis machine to clean our blood artificially.

Some chemicals can help our bodies detoxify by making our livers more efficient. One of them, for example, is sulforaphane. In 1992 researchers from John Hopkins University in Baltimore discovered that cruciferous vegetables and especially broccoli contained a substance referred to as glucoraphanin. It is a precursor to the natural antioxidant and cancer-inhibiting detoxifying isothiocyanate called sulforaphane. It is chemical that is present almost exclusively in cruciferous vegetables and with adequate levels only in fresh broccoli. Broccoli sprouts are the richest origin of glucosinolates and isothiocyanates that boost antioxidant status, induce phase 2 detoxification enzymes in the liver and protect animals against chemically induced cancer. Phase 1 enzymes activate or deactivate carcinogens. Phase 2 enzymes detoxify. For more than 20 years researchers had known that eating cruciferous vegtables induce enzyme detoxification in experimental studies. Isothiocyanate sulforaphane is identified as the principal phase 2 inducer in broccoli extracts. Sulforaphane is the most potent natural phase 2 enzyme-inducer know to science. It is also demonstrated that sulforaphane is a dose-related inhibitor of carcinogen-induced mammary tumorigenesis. So eat broccoli, but there is a catch, it must be raw and well chewed same as garlic. Also, broccoli sprouts contain 10–100 times the phase 2 inducer activity of mature broccoli plants. If we want to boost liver function adding raw broccoli sprouts to the salad is a good option. Supplement single-nutrient approaches to cancer prevention and detoxifying, and inflammation lowering have usually yielded worsening results. Isolated phytochemical approaches can be proven to be equally disappointing and are not recommended at least at the time being until supplemental sulforaphane is not thoroughly tested in double-blind studies on humans. So far broccoli extract which contains sulforaphane is tested with positive results. Alternatively, eat raw broccoli. In micromoles per gram mature broccoli has 64 of sulforaphane, the number two kohlrabi 28 and cauliflower 11. Broccoli raab is just 0.13 not even worth mentioning. While broccoli, broccolini, and Chinese broccoli are closely related to cabbage, the closest kin to broccoli rabe is turnips. Also, there is no sulforaphane in frizzed broccoli in cooked broccoli in steamed broccoli, and actually, there is none in raw broccoli as well. It is only formed when something bites the broccoli flower as a defensive mechanism. Sulforaphane is a natural pesticide for insects. The enzymes that create sulforaphane are heat sensitive but the sulforaphane itself is not. If we freeze or cook before we bite, there is nothing in it. The more we chew, the better and yes that is the taste that gives the broccoli bad raps. The same pesticide that forces the insects to spit the stuff out. Broccoli sprout taste is not that bad and can go nicely with little salad dressing or in a sandwich.

Our bodies have detoxifying enzymes not just in the liver but in the lungs and throat to help us deal with air pollutants directly before they enter the bloodstream. Some people are born with less active detox enzymes in the airways and have an allergic reaction to pollutants in the air like diesel exhaust and can have asthma attacks. These enzymes clean the pollutants from the air which enter our lungs and lowers the inflammation. The estimate was that 15-20 percent of the general population has some of the defective enzymatic function in air pathways making them prone to allergic reactions and asthma. Short-term ingestion of broccoli sprout homogenates has been shown to reduce nasal inflammatory responses to oxidant pollutants (Effect of 10-day broccoli consumption on inflammatory status of young healthy smokers. Int J Food Sci Nutr. 2014 Feb;65(1):106-11). There are the same enzymes in our air pathways that exist in the liver. So the sulforaphane increases the effectiveness of our lungs too not just the liver. C reactive protein (inflammation marker) can be elevated 20 years after quitting but with feeding people raw broccoli (250 grams a day) like in the above study plasma CRP level decreased 48% after ten days. In this one (Oral sulforaphane increases Phase II antioxidant enzymes in the human upper airway. Clin Immunol. 2009 Mar;130(3):244-51) they discovered that sulforaphane induces mucosal phase 2 enzyme expression in the upper airway of human subjects and confirms the effect phase 2 enzymes initiation in the airway as a method to decrease the inflammatory impacts of oxidative stress. How much more? About 100 times more detox enzyme expression. In this study in China (Rapid and sustainable detoxification of airborne pollutants by broccoli sprout beverage: results of a randomized clinical trial in China. Cancer Prev Res (Phila). 2014 Aug;7(8):813-823) which has the highest level of air pollution in the world broccoli extract increased the levels of excretion of the benzene by 61%, and acrolein by 23% (irritant for the skin, eyes, and nasal passages). There was concern that this level of lowering inflammation response might be dangerous because it might end up lowering our inflammation response to influenza viruses too. The studies that looked into this, showed no immune suppressive effect but completely the opposite, increasing immune effect besides lowering the inflammation. The best of both worlds. The bottom line is to eat the raw broccoli. Also, chew it well. If you want to you can add it in a green smoothie or blend it and let it sit there for some time and then use for something maybe soup. There was one study from the University of Reading that found the addition of raw powdered mustard seeds to the heat-processed broccoli significantly increased the formation of sulforaphane. Both the mustard and broccoli are from the same family of plants and have these enzymes. The researchers found out that adding a minor quantity of ground raw mustard seeds to the heat-processed broccoli significantly increased the formation of sulforaphane. The amount of sulforaphane that is formed in this way is almost identical to the amount that is formed when eating raw broccoli so if you do not dislike muster taste you can go for it. The myrosinase enzyme is found in mustard seeds in horseradish, wasabi powder or daikon radish.

There is one more scientifically proven way to lover toxin exposure if you are a woman. You can have a baby. You will transfer some of the toxins to the child. Some woman can halve their values of POPs during pregnancy. Firstborn children always have the highest levels of toxins leaving less for their brothers down the line. Toxin levels in breast milk also drop after the first pregnancy. If you do nothing, at least it would be a good idea to go healthy whole food vegan diet and detoxify as much as possible if you want to conceive at least for one year before pregnancy. Just quitting drugs, pills, alcohol, and smoking are not enough.